Jessica Cornwell is a writer living in Somerset. Born in California, she studied at Stanford and the Institute of Theatre in Barcelona before moving to London to work in film. Her first novel, *The Serpent Papers*, was published in 2015 to great acclaim. In 2018 she became the mother to twin boys. *Birth Notes* is her first work of non-fiction.

'An unflinchingly honest exploration of birth trauma, and ultimately a redemptive tale of the power and wisdom of women's bodies' Leah Hazard, author of *Womb: The Inside Story of Where We All Began*

'Vivid, beautiful and brave, this book undid me – and filled me with hope' Elinor Cleghorn, author of *Unwell Women*

'A hauntingly beautiful and unflinching, yet graciously shared experience of birth and motherhood. I savoured every word from the very first page' Abi Daré, author of *The Girl with the Louding Voice*

'Magnificent … a work of truth, understanding, scholarship and hope. A major contribution to women's experience' Susie Orbach, author of *In Therapy*

'An astonishing memoir. It is about the intersection between birth trauma and sexual trauma, medical misogyny, and trying to find a way to be a mother while dealing with something unspeakable. It is hugely important, courageous, and beautifully written. A rallying cry' Rhiannon Lucy Cosslett, author of *The Tyranny of Lost Things*

'A feat of strength. Jessica Cornwell doesn't shy away from the conflicting forces at work on women's bodies women will feel less alone aft Ward, author of *Girl Reading*

'Cornwell puts words to experiences that are often rendered beyond words because they are of traumas that are minimised, shamed or shunned. Her prose is presented with arresting beauty and I know her book speaks for countless others' Julia Bueno, author of *Everyone's a Critic*

'A riveting and deeply moving examination of birth trauma and post traumatic stress in a world where new mothers and their needs are too often ignored or dangerously minimised ... skilfully and beautifully written' Michelle Bowdler, author of *Is Rape a Crime? A Memoir, an Investigation and a Manifesto*

'A luminous, visceral reel of life after birth and trauma. At once devastating, validating, tender and raw, Cornwell guides us through the foundations of the hardest moments of her life with honesty and invitation ... I found it impossible to put down, her words endlessly comforting in their openness' Caitriona Morton, author of *How We Survive*

'Stunning ... This book will change lives, for it is a quest, a fight, a light, casting away hundred-years-old shadows. It is a book of love' Adélaïde Bon, author of *The Little Girl on the Ice Floe*

BIRTH NOTES

A Memoir of Trauma, Motherhood and Recovery

JESSICA CORNWELL

virago

VIRAGO

First published in Great Britain in 2022 by Virago
This paperback edition published in Great Britain in 2023 by Virago

1 3 5 7 9 10 8 6 4 2

A CIP catalogue record for this book
is available from the British Library.

Extracts on pages 385 to 387 from *I Am Not Your Baby Mother*
© Candice Brathwaite (London: Quercus, 2020) reproduced
with permission of the Licensor through PLSclear.

Paperback ISBN 978-0-349-014272

*In order to maintain anonymity in some instances,
the author has changed the names and identifying
features of certain individuals.*

Typeset in Sabon by M Rules
Printed and bound in Great Britain by Clays Ltd, Elcograf S.p.A.

Papers used by Virago are from well-managed forests
and other responsible sources.

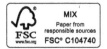

Virago
An imprint of
Little, Brown Book Group
Carmelite House
50 Victoria Embankment
London EC4Y 0DZ

An Hachette UK Company
www.hachette.co.uk

www.littlebrown.co.uk

For the others

The nurses give back my clothes, and an identity.
It is usual, they say, for such a thing to happen.
It is usual in my life, and the lives of others.

Sylvia Plath

SPRING

*A*s I write this, my boys are sleeping upstairs. I am thirty-three and they are twenty-five months old and it is naptime. I am sitting cross-legged in our rented living room, with a laptop on my knees surrounded by the chaos of toddlerhood: my twins' discarded beakers and soft toys, their cotton dribble bibs and beloved books, their blocks and wooden trains. I do not have an office. I work in stolen moments, whenever they are sleeping, mostly in the kitchen nursing a coffee or perched on this sofa, at the heart of my children's universe. It is always a balancing act: do I sweep the floor, run a load of laundry, clean their trays for the next meal or write a paragraph? I have a soup in the slow cooker, and their sweaters folded in neat piles, and my mask in my coat pocket, in case we go outside.

I have read, somewhere, that the first thousand days of an infant's life – from conception until their second birthday – are crucial in their development as a child. This is the story of the first thousand days of my development as a mother. I am an unreliable narrator. Memories are mutable and strange and what I remember, I cannot always be certain I remember exactly. But I have done my best, wherever possible, to tell the truth.

AFTERBIRTH

Time is short and full, like an outgrown frock.

Emily Dickinson

When the midwife pushed the fluid in, she whispered 'Shit' as the pressure of the needle blew everything out. I could recall, clearly, the pain, though the cause of it would remain confusing. Later, lying in my hospital bed, I'd watch the yellow bruising from this incident ripple up my skin like a scar.

My room on the postnatal* ward was painted a sickly mint, pastel and saccharine, like an ice cream. The cot for newborns, also mint green, lay empty at my bedside, and I had difficulty understanding why. The midwives came regularly, as regularly as they could. They took my temperature and measured my heart rate and blood pressure, and gave me compression socks to help with clotting and injections in the fat of my thighs.

---

*Puerperal, postnatal and postpartum refer to the same time period, the months immediately following childbirth, and are used synonymously throughout this text.

NHS maternity wards are communal. Beds line up like sardines, separated by thin, dingy curtains. But this was different. Mine was a small room, tucked away from other mothers with their newborns. The doors closed. I had a sink and a wardrobe and a bedside table. Such luxury came at a cost: this was the place mothers went when they had suffered. When they had been severed from their baby, and needed to be protected from witnessing what they did not have: an infant nuzzling on their breast. This was the room of still-births. Of children who came too early and slept alone in incubators. It was the room of women like me, who had met the cruel face of nature and survived. I was lucky. I had not lost my children, would not lose my children. But I had nearly lost my life and I did not have my babies with me, as the antibiotics dripped into my arm and I drifted in and out of consciousness, three weeks after my twins had been born.

Throughout, I fixated on the view from the mint-green room. Mostly it was grey and foggy and bleak, but when the clouds lifted, I could see pigeons roosting on a tiled roof and the exit of the parking lot where cars slipped in and out, bringing people in to visit patients, and taking patients home. I imagined myself in a car returning to my babies, wondering what this would be like, and when it would happen. Perhaps today? Perhaps tomorrow? I did not want the bacteria living in my womb to continue poisoning my body, so I was a good patient, well behaved. I did not hit the help button too many times or ask irritating questions in the night. I slept when they said I should sleep and did not move my arm when my veins collapsed from the treatment, and the cannula had to be relocated. There was a pleasant quality to the loneliness, something calm, as the fluids and the painkillers and the antibiotics dripped into my body. They would smile nicely and look at my vitals and say, 'You're doing well.' Not once in that process did a doctor or a midwife call me by my name, nor did I see the same doctor twice – but I barely noticed this anonymity. My namelessness reflected the place I had entered, with its bare green walls and plain white bed. I missed my children. When my breasts woke me in the night, bursting with liquid, I pumped in my room, sitting up on my bed, filling little plastic bottles with my milk like a dairy cow. I would take my IV apparatus, rattling on its rickety metal wheels, past the rows of sleeping mothers into the communal kitchen, pull off a label from a pad and inscribe my milk with my name and patient number, copying this from the laminated band I wore around my wrist. I would leave my milk in the fridge overnight, beside other little bottles. In the morning, members of my husband's family would come to collect this milk and deliver it to my children. I liked these visits, however brief. My milk, in the clinical sterile bottles, its purpose, its urgency, was my lifeline.

Inside the mint-green room, medicine stripped me down and cleaned me out, and for that I was very grateful. Only once was someone unkind to me. I emerged from a dreamless sleep and found that my nurse had forgotten to replace my medicine, and the bag that held the fluid and the antibiotics had emptied. My blood had begun to travel up through the needle, filling the empty bag, with a rapidity that alarmed me. I panicked and pressed the button urgently for help, and then when no one came, I got shakily out of bed, and left my room, still attached to the drip, taking my blood with me. I stumbled through the postnatal ward, seeking the midwives' desk, and when I arrived, desperate and on the verge of tears, I cried out, 'Make it stop!', insisting they take the needle out of my arm. Later, when the same midwife came to check my vitals and I apologised for being frightened, she snapped at me and said: 'You are traumatised.'

Was I traumatised?

I had given birth, vaginally, to twins at thirty-eight weeks, following an induction. I had a forceps and ventouse delivery with an emergency, manual extraction of my placentas. I had a haemorrhage, and a second degree tear, and an episiotomy. I lost 1.6 litres of blood. The doctor had inserted her arm into my womb blind and tugged out my twins' placentas with her fingers, leaving me filled with something she called *ragged membranes*. This doctor saved my life, but no one took the time to tell me why or how this had happened or what recovery would look like. Had I been sanguine enough to ask, perhaps someone might have explained my condition, but when the operating room emptied, I found myself alone with one child, incapable of saying a word. My husband had vanished with our second baby, a baby who I had first seen shooting through the operating-room doors wearing a blue mask as I bled out in a gathering crowd, without my husband, without my second child, surrounded by strangers, clasping my firstborn son to my chest until they took him away and the female anaesthetist, who was Spanish, held my head, saying, 'Talk to me. Look at me.' But I couldn't talk. I couldn't say anything at all. I looked into her eyes as the fluid rushed through my body, and strangers were pushing hard, on my belly, reaching up and in, trying to staunch the bleeding, and I looked at her, tears streaming down my cheeks, and thought: *You are beautiful.* I felt a tugging and a crunching and a pulling and a falling and then I was gone, somewhere very far away.

11

In the drug-induced fugue that followed, I dreamed fitfully. I returned to my parents' house in California. I sat at their kitchen table, looking through the window at warm, blue mountains. I saw the peach-coloured roses against stucco walls, and the dark fingers of cypress on our drive, and the thick wooded hills leading down to the valley. I visited each of my seven younger siblings, my adolescent brothers and sisters reading books in their rooms, the baby, twenty-one years younger than myself, playing beside the dog. That dog is dead now, hit by a car, but back then he was alive, and we lived in a house my parents built at the foothills of the Los Padres National Forest in Southern California. I dreamed of this house deeply, the way the morning light came through the windows, the way the citrus blossom perfumed the air in spring, the way the hummingbirds' wings flashed opalescent in the sun as they drank from our fountain. But then came the drought, and then came the Thomas Fire, and when I awoke after giving birth to two children, I had no childhood home to return to and no husband to hold my hand, and only one baby in the cot beside me.

I will remember this sensation for ever: the utter certainty that my second child had died. That he, like my home, had vanished. Burned up in the fire. Like the house, the trees, the fountain, he had gone, with every physical marker of my family's lifetime – every piece of art, every heirloom, every diary entry, every messy note left scribbled on the kitchen counter. When it came to my parents' house, what remained was startlingly apocalyptic: mangled walls, a burnt-out chimney containing the corpse of a coyote, the charred stumps of trees, the blackened, toxic earth. My teenage sister Catherine saw the fire first, through the kitchen window, loading the dishwasher on a warm December evening, Santa Ana winds blowing hard from the east. I woke, in London, to a text from my father, who sent a photograph of fire kindling beneath the moon, appearing on the ridgeline of a cloudless night. There was no formal evacuation, no warning. Forty minutes later, fire engulfed the house. My parents escaped with the clothes on their backs, their laptops and phones, and their animals, two dogs and four cats. My two youngest sisters were the only ones to gather anything personal: each packed a single bag of belongings in the minutes that they had, and they hold that they did this because they knew that the fire was absolute, that nothing would be left when it was over. The horse my family could not rescue, and had no time to do anything about other than leave him in a locked paddock. I remember my mother calling me that night, when I was pregnant, and crying about this horse. That she felt guilty. That she should have driven up there and opened the gate, no matter how close the fire was, that it was her fault that she had abandoned him to the blaze. He survived. His eyes, though, have darkened, and when I returned to visit him, almost a year later, I found a distant, anxious animal, forever changed by the inferno he had witnessed burning around him. This was a very strange time for my family.

I am not by nature a depressive person. When my parents' house burned down, three months before I gave birth, I cried for a day and felt better. No one had died and a house was just a material thing, full of material objects. My parents had insurance, they would rebuild, the rain would come, the aquifers would fill, the trees would grow back, the animals return. I had an indomitable belief in possibility that came from a place of power and whiteness and privilege. Maggie Nelson writes: 'Privilege *saturates*. Privilege *structures*.' Nothing makes privilege more abundantly apparent than witnessing myriad consequences – and sobering inequalities – of natural disaster. My father, an Emmy award-winning film producer, the son of a famous novelist, came from a wealthy, creative family. Yes, the house, the possessions, had been lost, but, economically speaking at least, the family would be fine. When I submitted a partial manuscript masquerading as a book, a few days after the house burned down, and my publisher sensibly rejected it, this too was fine. I was an optimist. Optimism was a personal philosophy: a way of being. Before motherhood, I had never had therapy, or been diagnosed with depression. I had never, or so I lied to myself, experienced anxiety. I had moved from one elite academic institution to another in a way that was entitled and unflappable. I was a gilded overachiever with a positive attitude. When I felt my children kicking in my womb, and put my hand to my belly to greet them, I basked in the self-satisfied glow of pregnancy. Books and houses? They would come and go. There were other, more important things in life: my family. My future. My children. My loved ones.

At the hospital of my children's birth, I had a catheter and a bedpan. I could not move from my bed without fainting, needed assistance in the shower. I struggled to walk or stand, I had lost so much blood following my labour that this compounded my anaemia, leaving me woozy and uncertain. My hair darkened, my skin became translucent, almost grey, all colour drained from my cheeks. My mood improved after a blood transfusion, but this arrived late at my bedside, as the haemorrhage I had suffered was not recorded in the midwives' notes. After fainting, bloodwork revealed I was anaemic, and units were called for ... but still, delays. The blood was lost, then found, then lost again. When the units finally arrived, the wrong type came, a mistake I caught when the midwife held the label up for me to read, before being attached to the drip, and the little dance of waiting began again. After delivery, the high-dependency unit was full, and certain information had been mislaid. I was sent instead to the postnatal ward, where the majority of midwives were overstretched and unhappy. Most did not like to change cannulas or administer transfusions. On the second day in bed, still waiting for the units, the midwife on the ward told me I could not have the blood that evening, though it had arrived. This, she explained – she was pretty and Irish and had a rakish lilt – was because she was managing twenty-nine patients alone and she did not have the expertise or the time to help me with my condition. In the beginning, I hated this woman; I thought her draconian and cruel. Later, when I heard her crying in the corridor, I realised she too was trapped in a system which was breaking her, and that there was nothing, really, anyone could do.

After delivery, I did not meet my second son. I was too sick to see him, and he was too sick to see me, so instead I pumped colostrum from my breast and sent this with my husband to the Neonatal Intensive Care Unit, where our son was on CPAP, and being treated for an infection. As I recovered, my husband gave our son skin-to-skin in the NICU, and fed him through a little tube. He ran back and forth between us like a messenger, returning with stories of our son's IV, his drip and antibiotics, saying that they were worried for a while, but he was doing better. Alone, in the postnatal ward, without my husband, with one infant when I was meant to have two, I struggled. Breastfeeding felt violent and difficult. Neither Baby A nor I knew anything about it. I was too weak to hold my child up, and because my husband was not there to help, a kind nurse came and spoke to me, and, on condition that I promise not to tell the midwives, she held my breast in place and helped the baby latch, and stayed by my side until she was satisfied that he was drinking, despite how busy she was, patting my arm and saying, 'You're a strong woman.'

Throughout my stay in hospital, three other strong women occupied the hospital bed across from me. The first was a young Greek mother, attended by her husband and doula. With the doula's guidance, an atmosphere of serenity formed around the newborn child. The parents were quiet *in extremis*. Even to the midwives they whispered. The formation of bodies, around the baby, was sacred, near-biblical, like a Caravaggio painting. Their stillness touched me.

The second woman to convalesce across from me was English, and horsey, and loud. Her husband lounged on the hospital bed, shirtless, reading his mobile phone, complaining of being tired, while she struggled in the chair beside him, trying to get her baby to latch. That evening, when the husband went home to rest, the mother was friendly from the bed, she smiled. Of her baby, she said, 'My husband wants to name it Pan.' Why Pan? She told a story about a statue of a faun they had seen on an Italian holiday and shuddered: she had never liked *Pan,* preferred Peter. As to her own body? Forceps, tear. 'But we all muck on, don't we?' she said, not sounding in the least convinced.

The third woman was a petite Ethiopian lady of profound elegance. After she had curled beside her newborn, her husband kissed her and returned home to gather the older children. When he left, she came over, while her baby slept, to look at the twins. 'What happened to you?' she asked, watching the blood enter my arm. 'I don't know,' I said. 'I can't remember.' On arrival, her children embraced their mother, joyously, clamouring around her, eager to hold the new baby. The husband came again to our bedside, offering a bowl of *genfo*, a traditional porridge made for mothers after birth. 'Eat this,' he said, looking at the blood-encrusted cannula taped dirtily to my hand. 'It will restore your strength.' I ate. The porridge, like the transfusion, was thick and nourishing.

There was another, too, among us, obscured by the curtained chambers of our ward. She remained veiled throughout, but at night, I heard her praying. At night, I heard her muttering. At night, I heard her crying. In the morning, a specialist assessed her. The mother told the specialist that she was seeing things. Lots of things. A serpent, slithering about the room. She had visions. Of dying children. Of children who sucked poison from breasts. Of children who were, themselves, serpents. Of children who brought bad luck. The specialist told the mother that they had taken her baby into care. The specialist asked if there was anyone at home, anyone who would like to be here now, anyone who could help her, before the mother herself was institutionalised. 'No,' the mother said. 'No'. Her *No*, in its absoluteness, its aloneness, struck me.

It struck me hard.

A woman is a ritual

reads a fragment of Genny Lim's 1981 poem 'Wonder Woman':

A house that must accommodate
A house that must endure

In 1959, the Italian anthropologist and historian Ernesto de Martino published *Sud e magia,* a study of ceremonial magic and witchcraft in Southern Italy. Of the binding rituals practised by women after childbirth, he observed:

In Lucania, there is a widely documented relationship between the placenta and milk. In Savoia, a woman dips the placenta several times in a river, accompanying the gesture with this formula:

come se jegne sta borza	(Just as this bag gets filled with
d'acqua	water
cussí se pozzano anghí sti menne	so may these breasts be filled with
de latte.	milk)

She repeats the formula three times and finishes with an Our Father. In Pisticci, a stone holds down the umbilical cord and placenta in the middle of a stream, so that the water flows over them at length and the placenta gets filled with it. In Viggiano and in Valsinni, to reinforce the magical operation, a small piece detached from the placenta left in the stream may be used to prepare a broth for the mother.

My mother's people were Lucanian. In the winter of 1903, my maternal great-grandfather, Donato Vona, then three years old, walked with his mother from the woods of Monte Vulture to Naples, where he boarded a ship to New York, 'a stowaway beneath his mother's skirts', or so my Uncle Patrick tells it. After birth, I considered this woman, seeking a better life for her son, and wondered if she practised rituals in the Old Country, washing her placenta clean in the river.

Bedbound, in hospital, guided by algorithms, soothed by the silent glow of my phone, I stumbled across an article on my phone from *parents.com* titled: 'Celeb moms who ate their placentas'. Chrissy Teigen did it, and January Jones did it, and Katherine Heigl, and Tia and Tamera Mowry, and Mayim Bialik, and Gaby Hoffmann (*'Placenta, placenta, placenta,* Hoffmann told *People* magazine, *just eat that sh*t up, and it does a girl good'*). Though I had never, personally, wished to eat my placenta, I found these celebrities' approach to birth and their body refreshingly radical, refreshingly magical. Kim Kardashian famously ate her own placenta to avoid postpartum depression after giving birth to her second child. *I'm having it freeze-dried and made into a pill form,* she shared on her app, *not actually fry it like a steak and eat it (which some people do, BTW).*

Kim did this because she had suffered a rare and dangerous complication called placenta accreta in both pregnancies.

My doctor had to stick his entire arm in me and detach the placenta with his hand, Kim blogged in 2015, describing her first child North's birth, *scraping it away from my uterus with his fingernails. How disgusting and painful!!! My mom was crying; she had never seen anything like this before. My delivery was fairly easy, but then going through that – it was the most painful experience of my life!*

For Kim, eating her placenta, the second time round, was positive: *Every time I take a pill*, she wrote, *I feel a surge of energy and feel really healthy and good. I totally recommend it for anyone considering it!*

Mary Wollstonecraft gave birth to her second daughter, Mary Shelley, at midnight on Wednesday, 30 August 1797, attended by the midwife Mrs Blenkinsop. The baby was healthy, but the placenta would not dislodge. Hours passed. Increasingly worried, the midwife alerted Mary's husband, Mr Godwin, who in turn summoned a doctor who in turn inserted his hand into Wollstonecraft's womb, ripping out her placenta. Like Kim, Mary told her husband that the procedure was the most excruciating of her life. A few days later, Mary woke and complained of chills. Fever followed. She died shortly thereafter. Mr Godwin experienced such intense grief that he was unable to attend her funeral.

My own placenta, gouged out in pieces, was carried away in a white plastic bowl after birth and carefully reassembled, before being disposed of in hospital waste. This fragmented placenta-in-absentia increasingly upset me. Maybe I should have demanded it back, like Kim Kardashian. Maybe I should have eaten it. Maybe if I had participated in a mystical act of self-consumption, I would understand what had happened to my body. Maybe I would not be so tired, so weak, so bloodless, so confused.

'Placentophagy', the eating of the placenta, is widespread among mammals postpartum, but it is not, technically speaking, widespread among the human population. *The American Journal of Obstetrics and Gynecology* published an expert review of Human Placentophagy in April 2018. The review concluded:

> Without any scientific evidence, individuals promoting placentophagy, especially in the form of placenta encapsulation, claim that it is associated with certain physical and psychosocial benefits. We found that there is no scientific evidence of any clinical benefit of placentophagy among humans, and no placental nutrients and hormones are retained in sufficient amounts after placenta encapsulation to be potentially helpful to the mother postpartum. In contrast to the belief of clinical benefits associated with human placentophagy, the Centers for Disease Control and Prevention recently issued a warning due to a case in which a newborn infant developed recurrent neonatal group B Streptococcus sepsis after the mother ingested contaminated placenta capsules containing Streptococcus agalactiae. The Centers for Disease Control and Prevention recommended that the intake of placenta capsules should be avoided owing to inadequate eradication of infectious pathogens during the encapsulation process.

Several Californian friends of mine had eaten their placentas. Where they had not eaten them, they had planted them ceremonially under trees.

On the sixth day in hospital, well enough to walk, at last, to the maternity ward's cafeteria, I encountered a father, distraught, at reception. 'What do you mean, you've lost it?' he shouted at the woman behind the desk. 'We asked you to keep her placenta safe. We asked you to give it back to us.'

Simone de Beauvoir argued in *The Second Sex* that:

> pregnancy is above all a drama playing itself out in the woman between her and herself. She experiences it both as an enrichment and a mutilation; the foetus is part of her body and it is a parasite exploiting her; she possesses it and she is possessed by it; it encapsulates the whole future and in carrying it, she feels as vast as the world; but this very richness annihilates her, she has the impression of not being anything else. A new existence is going to manifest itself and justify her own existence, she is proud of it; but she also feels like the plaything of obscure forces, she is tossed about, assaulted.

Perhaps the placenta is a locus of the 'obscure forces' that assault a woman in birth. Perhaps by consuming her placenta, the mediating organ between mother and child, a woman may feel, after birth, that she has reasserted dominion over her own body. That she has controlled what was once uncontrollable. Inspired by the man at reception, I decided to ask the midwives what had happened to my own missing placenta. Why had it been ripped out like that? Why did I lose so much blood? Why did it hurt so badly, deep inside me? Together, with my husband Callum, we consulted the notes. *Normal vaginal delivery*, the notes read. *No complications*. But that's wrong, Callum retorted, becoming nearly as irate as the man I had seen in reception. She had an induction, he said, pointing at me. She had complications. 'I'm sorry,' a midwife said, scribbling her own corrections in the margin. 'Somebody must have made a mistake.'

On the evening of the seventh day, Callum and I left hospital, carrying the sleeping twins in their car seats proudly across the threshold of our maisonette apartment, and together began the all-important work of parenting.

The night I first fell ill – truly, badly, deeply ill, after the birth of my children – I told Callum I felt cold. Strangely cold. My heart was beating rapidly in my chest, so rapidly that I was scared, and I said, somewhat hysterically, that I was afraid I was going to die. Callum reassured me gently that this was not going to happen. That I was tired and perhaps I was experiencing something similar to a panic attack. I grew angry, and withdrew. Later that evening, he apologised, suggesting I take a bath while the twins slept. 'You should relax,' he said. This I also remember clearly: him touching my arm and saying, 'Relax, leave them with me, the babies. They will be fine; I will keep an eye on them.' And then myself, wandering downstairs, extremely slowly, holding on to the banister, worried that I might fall. After that? Nothing. I must have had a bath, because I woke, briefly, naked, on the floor, wrapped in a white towel, and I could feel somebody's hands on me and hear the buzzing of a space heater, and the hot air on my body, and I remember repeating that I was cold. In the delirium that followed, I recall my mother's face, very close to mine, and that she spoke my name as she sat on our bed in our little home. She put her hand to my forehead as she had done when I was a child, and said to my husband that I was hot, too hot, and together they agreed that he should take me back to hospital. I cried and begged them not to, saying I did not want to go back, not to that place where I had been interred with my children.

At hospital, a female midwife and female doctor, whose names and faces I do not remember, took my blood and examined my cervix and said that I was sick. My uterus was infected and I had the beginning of sepsis. The cannulas returned, and the little shunt entered my left hand, perhaps the ninth, perhaps the tenth time in the twenty-odd days since the babies had been born.

The midwife pushing the fluid in whispered 'Shit' as the pressure of the needle killed the vein.

Later, lying in my hospital bed, I would watch yellow bruising from the incident ripple up my skin like a scar.

Judith Herman, *Trauma and Recovery*, 1992:

Psychological trauma is an affliction of the powerless.
At the moment of trauma, the victim is rendered helpless
by overwhelming force. When the force is that of nature,
we speak of disasters. When the force is that of other
human beings, we speak of atrocities. Traumatic events
overwhelm the ordinary systems of care that give people
a sense of control, connection, and meaning.

But what is it when the force is that of childbirth?

Primipara. That's what they called me. *A woman giving birth for the first time. Past/Present/Future/Now.* Novice. Neophyte. New. 'Does this hurt?' the doctor asked the next morning, doing the rounds, standing above me. There it goes again: the flickering. The living between multiple planes at once. The old, familiar numbness. Rather than examining me internally, the man grinds his fingers into the flesh of my lower abdomen, hunting for pain. 'Does this hurt?' he asks again. 'No,' I say, exiting my body. 'Nothing hurts.' The doctor frowns, pushing again harder, pressing his fingers into my pelvis, my stomach, my groin, and when I do not scream, and stare blankly into space, unmoved, he snaps, to my husband, to the assembled others, 'There's been a mistake. She shouldn't be here.' He says, 'If she had anything in there,' he gestures to my womb, 'she would have screamed. She would have jumped a mile.' The medical notes, written by this man, read: *No sign of suspected uterine infection.*

I am sick today, sick in my body, writes Japanese poet Yosano Akiko (1878–1942) in 'Labour Pains', a poem in which a pleasant young doctor describes the joy of giving birth to a woman who has given birth before, and the labouring woman, the narrator of the poem, takes strength in her own self-knowledge:

Since I know better than he about this matter,
what good purpose can his prattle serve?

At home, things exited me. Blood first, in small quantities, then large, globular streaks of tissue, purple and shiny. Then fingers of flesh, pale pink, with an ugly greenish sheen, grey at the edges, and a putrid smell, like old meat left out too long on the counter. Each time I went to the bathroom, each time I wiped myself and smelled that awful, rancid smell, I understood, on some animal level, that my body had become a festival of decay, that I was rotting, gently, from the inside out. In the morning, I sobbed over the toilet, showing Callum the worst of it, the mottled carnage slough-ing out of me, fouling the water, thickening the tissue, as he soothed a crying baby in his arms. 'Oh, God,' he said, and went very quiet and helped me back into bed, and handed me the babies to feed and called another hospital, a short drive from our home, the hospital with the mint-green room, where I was admitted, less than twenty-four hours after the consultant had discharged me, for a uterine infection, caused by 'retained products of conception' (retained pieces of placenta), and cared for by new and different midwives, on a new and different ward, over new and different days.

Convalescing in the mint-green room, I entered a blankness that did not lift. The antibiotics left a metallic taste in my mouth I couldn't stomach, but this was about the only sensory thing I noticed. Outside of recognising physical discomfort, I couldn't laugh, couldn't cry, couldn't dream. I struggled to empathise, to understand what was happening around me; I felt no warmth, no joy, no love. I knew abstractly that I ought to feel these things. That I *once had* felt these things. That I *needed* to feel these things – for my children's sake, for my family's, for my own – but now, in this moment, I felt nothing. Birth shattered me, cutting through my world like a knife, severing all sense of connection. I fought hard against the symptoms, as best I could.

Returning from hospital to my babies, I went through the motions. I put my infants to my breast, held them in place and felt nothing. I wrapped them gently in swaddling, laid them down to rest, and stared into a void. My husband had returned to work, and in hospital I had become a shell, an automaton mother, suspended in nothingness – a state of shock. The only thing I recognised was a terrible and constant dread that something fatal would befall my family. For weeks, I would not leave the house except to come back into hospital. I refused to bathe my children, convinced that one of them would drown. I would not go outside because I was frightened that a car would ride up on the kerb and kill us. That the stroller would hurtle out of my grip and crash into a wall, that a branch would fall from the tree and crush us, that bacteria in bottles would infect my babies, that one of my babies would cease to breathe, silently, in their sleep, and I would wake and find their little corpse in the morning and be unable to do anything. Beyond this acute paranoia, emotional experience of any kind entirely left me.

I had lived through numbness like this once before, when I was a child. One morning, when I was thirteen, I woke up to find half of my face had frozen. It was as if someone had taken a marker and drawn a line down my meridian. On one side, my face was completely normal. But on the other? I couldn't move my mouth, couldn't blink my eye, couldn't taste food on that side of my tongue. My parents rushed me to the doctors, where they diagnosed a condition called Bell's palsy, an unusual ailment in children. They said that in the night, I had suffered a minor stroke or a virus – or perhaps Lyme disease? – and some mysterious swelling in my skull had caused damage or trauma to a facial nerve, shutting off my brain's communication to half my face. I went to bed fine, and woke up disfigured. It was unclear how long this palsy would last. Soon after, a burning rash erupted in my ear, like a biblical plague. The doctors examined the bloody pustules and dark red scabs and came to the conclusion that this was, in fact, a rare neurological disorder called Ramsay Hunt syndrome. I stopped going to school, wore an eye-patch to protect the eye that could no longer blink, and took steroids. Because my mother was managing my care, and her tendency has always been towards Eastern medicine, she arranged a course of acupuncture, medical tinctures and herbal supplements. My palsy lasted several months. One of the lingering memories of this period is the sensation of numbness affecting the left side of my face. You could have driven a needle through that cheek and I would not have felt a thing. My experience of returning from hospital was identical. But this time, instead of affecting half my face, the numbness spread through my heart, like a poison.

I think, in retrospect, of fairy tales, of how characters cannot move forward without paying a heavy price – without giving up their eyes or flesh or blood – that they must undergo a ritual sacrifice to reach a happy ending.

For a long time following the birth of my children, I believed I was hysterical. That I had been struck down by some terrible ailment of antiquity, which the Hippocratic authors in the fourth century BC referred to as a *suffocating womb* or *hysterike pnix*. The womb taking on a silencing effect, travelling up and up and up, lodging itself, like a cork, in the throat. A perfidious disease of body and mind that rendered its sufferers mute. Best managed, according to the Ancients, with suppositories of sulphur and honey and aromatic pessaries, or fumigations of lampwick mixed with wine, barley, straw, tamarind and deer horn. *Hysterike pnix* evolved into what became known in the nineteenth century as hysteria, and hysteria suited me: it was, as far as I was concerned, the only logical outcome of a birth experience like mine. My uterus, after all, had been infected. Things hurt, badly, deep inside me, and I had become, as it were, a woman possessed. I felt I had discovered, through birth, a Foucauldian dialectic in which madness and non-madness, like mother and child, were *inextricably involved: inseparable at the moment when they do not yet exist, and existing for each other, in relation to each other, in the exchange which separates them.*

The doctors of ancient Greece rooted mental illness in the body, and studied the somatic causes of postpartum depression, connecting the foul-smelling vapours emitted by the womb after birth to clouds of melancholy enveloping the mind. Wombs were sticky, viscous, smoky, dark, and so too the depression that followed birth, blood-bound, they suggested, caused by a dangerous aberration in female biology – the over-production of lochial discharge: the blood, mucus and uterine tissue that emerges from the uterus after birth. In melancholic mothers, lochial discharge, suppressed after birth, became a flood, surging upwards in the body, filling every organ, until the uterine blood engulfed the mother's brain, resulting in agitation, delirium, attacks of mania. After birth, my womb remained mysteriously viscous. The cause equally opaque. Oral antibiotics worked for as long as I was on them, but as soon as one course finished the fever was back, and the cycle of infection continued, first for weeks, then for months. Each time the fever returned, my hysteria deepened, until very soon there were no books and there were no people. Or, at least, there were only two: my husband and my mother-in-law. They came and sat beside me. They spoke and I tried to listen. But I was always in pain and always enveloped in my children: a pillow strapped around my chest, my breasts swollen, exposed, the babies lying prostrate, pinned in place by the pillow, scrambling up towards the bulbous breast, biting at the nipple. I, fixing the babies, one after the other, held them steady with each hand. As they latched, their tiny mouths exploded with milk, they turned their heads, they screamed.

What was I to do? I had become a freak show. I had moved into a liminal place without language, defined by unutterable and expansive numbness and the babies clamped to my breasts. Without words, the days sped by. Metamorphosis was a state we embodied purely, mother and children, but I did not find it beautiful. I found it frightening and chaotic and cruel. In motherhood, I ceased to be what I had known before: becoming, instead, a beast. I grew sad and distant. I knew only my children and my confusion and the feudal nature of my task. I did not engage in reading, or ideas, or films, or public debate, or the internet, or gossip. I did not write anything down. As a result, I cannot now look back and say with any certainty on which day such and such an event occurred, just as I cannot remember precisely when my children first smiled, or first pressed up on their arms and knees, or reached out or cooed, or sat and held their heads up, boldly, on their own, or ate puréed vegetables, or uttered their first primeval syllable, 'da'. *Da. Da. Da.* I do not know these things because I did not record them. I did not record them, because after the birth of my children, I transcended the passing of time and existed only in an endless nothingness, in which the days themselves seemed to last a thousand hours. In this place, I was not present enough to take joy in the unfolding miracle of my children's existence, though I was present enough to ensure that they remained alive.

During the day, while my children slept and I was sick, I would lie awake and watch them breathe. On the internet, before they had been born, I had read that small babies (and mine were very small), were more likely to die of cot death, so I made myself their keeper, and guarded them, prone and vigilant. Ready in case they choked or gasped, or their heads lolled awkwardly to the side, cutting off their breath. I never slept when they slept: instead, I lay beside them on the bed and often leaned in and touched them, moving their swaddling or putting my finger to their lips to check their breathing. I would rest my palm, lightly, on their chests, and feel their bellies rise; my own breath would quicken, and I would turn away from them and stare at the ceiling. Minutes, or an hour, would go by, and I would check again. It was a compulsive, paranoid act: a gesture I repeated, again and again and again. Sometimes their breathing would grow so soft and so subtle as to disappear, and sensing this, I would reach into my children's cots and swoop them into my arms and hold them. The babies, rightly, would scream in indignation at my senseless disturbance of their peace and I would whisper to them then, heart racing, 'I am sorry, I am sorry, I am sorry', and hug them tight. In consolation, I would offer them my breasts and they would nurse, and in feeding them, I would feel the muscles of my heart unclench, for in feeding they were alive, and I had once again defeated death.

After birth, death, whom I'd narrowly escaped, came to visit often. Together, we observed the babies closely. We studied them through the gauzy netting of their cots, for hours on end, and as I came to know death, time expanded exponentially and I discovered two opposing states of being. The first was a sensation of extreme stasis: the impossibility of progression, the absence of a future. The second was a conviction of sudden and impending doom. Even if I'd had the words, I could not speak of such things, so I hid these feelings as best I could. Lying in the arms of death, beside my sleeping babies, I would study my children and then shift my body slightly and gaze at the hanging light attached to the ceiling by the window. The shutters of the room were white and slatted, and the evening sun made shadows on the floor. The timelessness, the sleeplessness, the endless feeding, the endless fear, the minutiae of growth exhibited in my babies, the constant narrowing of death: all were contained in this room and all overtook me.

'Be happy,' they said. Taking a baby from a cot, they would sit at the end of the bed, and tell me, encouragingly, when my body grew stronger and I looked less pale, to 'take stock'. To 'count your blessings'. To 'focus on the good'. To 'celebrate living'.

'Be grateful,' they said. 'You have your children.'

Gratitude, apparently, was meant to help.

My name had gone on a prayer list at the church. Be grateful for what? Were they blind to the truth? The present, as I witnessed it, was unforgiving. Nature, as I had witnessed it, was unforgiving. Motherhood, as I had witnessed it, was unforgiving. The room, as I had witnessed it, was unforgiving.

'Oh, hun,' Kasi said over the telephone, 'this is bad.' Kasi had recently moved to New York, after leaving a start-up that had been bought for a tidy sum in Silicon Valley and enrolling as a graduate student at the Columbia Journalism School. Kasi was the first person I told when I found out we were having twins, a month after my honeymoon, and the first person I spoke to honestly when I emerged, numb and confused, from the mint-green room in North London. 'Don't worry,' she said, 'I'm coming.' True to her word, she booked a last-minute flight and, seventy-two hours later, appeared in the doorway of my apartment, fresh from Manhattan, tall and beautiful as ever, blonde hair swept into a sporty pony-tail, brown Longchamp over her shoulder, a compact carry-on by her side, of a kind used by tech entrepreneurs. She embodied, in that moment, precisely the person you want in emergencies: feisty, immaculate, hyper-intelligent, a millennial Mary Poppins. I'd asked her not to ring the doorbell, terrified the twins would wake.

'Okay,' she whispered at the door, and hugged me. 'I'm here. Debrief. Tell me everything. No secrets.'

I focused immediately on what all new parents fixate on: sleep. Or rather, lack of it. Managing two newborns, I confessed to Kasi, was what religious men meant by purgatory. Suddenly, I had a messy life, full of nappies and milk bottles and sick-stained muslins. We had not slept, my husband and I, for weeks. He'd started work as a script editor at the

BBC, and needed to be on set at all hours, often from dawn to deep into the evening. While I was in hospital with my infection, Callum was with the babies, working shifts with his mother and brothers and sister, feeding our children my breast milk from bottles. He then had to go into work in the morning, often on only one or two hours' sleep. I do not know how he survived this, or kept his job. Now that I had returned from hospital, I felt I barely saw Callum, other than during the endless nocturnal waking, lying weakly in bed as he passed me first one baby, then the other, giving in to the emptiness as they feasted on me. Because they were small babies, with small tummies, on different schedules, my children fed constantly, day and night. Their appetites deep, their anxiety profound. I would curl round them, keeping them in little cots attached to the bed, separated by a thin screen, to prevent them from falling out, or me from rolling over them. Their sleep was not synchronised, and they woke in cycles, latched and fed, the pattern starting again – obliterating any hope of peace.

Kasi shifted her weight beside me, coltish, agitated.

'I bet as a baby, it's great to have one of these.' She poked my enormous tummy. 'It's like a built-in cushion for nursing.'

This was the signature sense of humour that had so irritated my mother when we were teenagers. Kasi was infamous in my family for a quality of honesty that made her (in my opinion) utterly remarkable; an attribute my mother, rather less sympathetically, referred to as *gaucheness*. We met when we were fourteen, at one of the most elite private boarding schools on the West Coast (now unhappily mired in a sexual misconduct scandal spanning forty years), in the foothills of my childhood valley. She a boarder: scathingly irreverent, a scholarship girl, the daughter of a fisherman, a born fighter.

I a day student: bookish, self-important, privileged, who went home every day to five younger siblings and a pregnant mother, managing an eccentric, feline-ridden household. (My mother had, at the time, taken on twenty-eight foster cats.) The boarding school allotted places for only four local students a year – two girls and two boys who attended at a 'discounted' rate – and these places were fought over bitterly by the wealthy of Ojai. I applied, on bed rest, during the recovery from my palsy, after reading Ernest Shackleton's account of his voyage to the South Pole. My parents were perplexed by my desire to attend this school. 'Why?' they asked. 'You won't fit in.' One of the cats, perhaps sensing my parents' unease, peed on my paper application the night before it was due. My mum dried it out on a heater. I remember handing this application in to the admissions office, in person, wearing my eye-patch, terrified they would detect the festering aroma of cat urine on the pages. Freshman year, I learned very quickly that in any conflict you wanted Kasi on your side. She would punch harder than anyone else – but she was also tremendously loyal and kind. A zero bullshit person, Kasi believed that the easiness I had experienced in my life made me sheltered and entitled, and she pointed this out wherever possible, with a wry, endearing fondness.

'You would say that,' she'd cut me off, 'but your background is not normal', making it clear I'd lost touch with reality. When we graduated from high school, I'd gotten into Stanford, and she'd been offered a place at a liberal arts college on the east coast. We took a year off – me to travel with a boyfriend, she to intern in the Midwest on the Kerry campaign. My relationship fell apart, John Kerry lost. We returned to California and worked local jobs for a winter. It was then that we hatched a plan to move to Spain. We applied to a language course at the University of Salamanca, and showed up in Madrid, with two battery-powered translators. Neither of us spoke a word of Spanish. We had home-stays – mine with a ninety-year-old and her daughter and Kasi's with a wife-beating father and a woman with a split lip. We assessed our environments, called each other from snowy payphones, and met in a café. 'Screw this,' Kasi said, when I got there, regaling me with a vivid account of the bruises on her host-mother's face, and the atmosphere in the house. 'We find a place together. Now.'

I told the old ladies, as politely as I could, that I was moving out and went with Kasi, the next morning, to get her suitcase. Kasi was not lying about the state of that marriage. We ate a sandwich together in Salamanca's central plaza, bought a map and two basic cell phones, went to the school registrar and set about finding a flat. We paid for a short-term let, sharing a room in an apartment populated by German graduate students, before eventually breaking out on our own. On our first adventure to a student club night, Kasi disappeared with a flamenco dancer from Madrid. I was petrified and spent the night waiting up for her, unable to reach her cell phone. She flounced in the next morning, with two lollipops as a peace offering, and told me not to worry. When the term ended, she went to Washington, and I went to Palo Alto. We missed each other hugely and Kasi wasn't happy. She came for a weekend in Palo Alto, and with Kasi-ish determination decided on a new course of action. She applied as a transfer student to my university and got in. We celebrated, championing her success loudly. But proximity, we soon discovered, did not make for easy friendship. We were too busy finding ourselves in our early twenties. Each competitive in our own way, each confronting our own problems, we struggled to be kind to each other, arguing over choices and values. But ours was the sort of friendship that weathered storms, and each time we came back, we came back closer.

'I wish I could say they were cute,' Kasi said, standing over the little cots. She paused before passing judgement. 'But I'm sure they will be one day.'

She was right: my babies weren't cute. They were tiny and weird and animal.

Finally, I thought, an objectively sane person has come to visit.

'What's it like being a mother?' she asked.

We were both looking at them.

I lied.

I said it was wonderful.

I couldn't admit to her, not then, that my primary emotion was one of shame. That my interactions with my children, while seeming tender, were utilitarian: not gestures of affection at all.

As I answered her questions, I recalled, privately, my first unnerving encounter with shame on the postnatal ward following the birth of my twins. This must have occurred before my blood transfusion, I think it was the evening of the second day, when Baby B returned in a trolley from the NICU and all four of us were reunited, on the public ward, for the first time, as a family. I was too weak to stand, so Callum passed me my newborn son while his brother slept in the clear plastic cot by my bedside, and I held my child against my breast. We had not named them yet, and so I used the old system, *in utero* this was Baby B – and despite being much smaller than I had imagined, his weight on my stomach hurt. Callum had told me very little about what he had seen of Baby B in the NICU, but he had described doing something called Kangaroo Care, and I had known better than to ask him too much. A year later, on the eve of celebrating their first birthdays, Callum broke down and wept. He told me of the blue mask our baby had worn, when they hooked him to the CPAP machine; of the fluid in his lungs that impacted his breathing; of the narrow plastic feeding tube inserted into his throat, taped to his cheek; of the cannula in his vein, delivering intravenous antibiotics; of his knitted hat, white with blue stripes, donated by charity, and the little square blanket, a patchwork quilt of coloured blocks, which he arrived with from the NICU. None of this I had seen, none of this I understood. Until a year later, when Callum mustered the courage to describe our sons' initial difficulties. The sound of A's resuscitation after birth, his uneven, laboured breathing, of all the things that had happened – things Callum deliberately hid on the second shared day of parenthood.

I had not seen our son in the NICU, but I saw the purple welt on his hand where the cannula had been. Baby B was sleeping when Callum handed him to me – and I could tell at once how much smaller Baby B was than his brother, wearing minute clothes, donated on the ward, and the white and blue knitted hat. The hat on B's head bothered me – it seemed evidence that something was wrong and so I removed it and felt my soul exit my body. As my husband marvelled at the tiny clothes they had given our son in the special care unit, telling me what a fighter he was – what a survivor! – all I could see was my son's deformed skull, the two egg-shaped wounds, purple and swollen – testimony to my child's unbearable vulnerability. I had failed him. He had spent his first two days alone in the NICU, without contact from his mother. I felt a great winding wave of shame: my child had needed me. I had been elsewhere. How could I protect this tiny being if I could not even muster the strength to be wheeled to his side? 'How did this happen?' I asked. Callum explained, very softly, that intervention during delivery had caused Baby B to haemorrhage on his skull at birth, and he now had what the midwives called a *double cephalohematoma*. The doctors promised it would go away, over time, but all I could think was: *I have done this. I have hurt my child.*

'It will get better,' Callum said. 'Focus on the good things: he's alive. He's alive and you're alive, and we're all here together now.'

Baby B woke and cried for a long time. I put my son to my breast, but my breast dwarfed him and he struggled to latch. A midwife came and helped, and once he had settled at the breast and drunk his fill, he relaxed into the place where my breast touched the crook of my arm and he let out a little exhale of satisfaction. I only realised then, that I was crying.

'I think we ought to introduce them,' Callum said. He took Baby B from me and laid him down in the shared cot beside his brother. I watched, stunned, blinking away tears, as the twins turned towards each other slowly, like plants following the sun, and squeaked at each other, feeling each other's fingers and eyes and mouth and nose with great tenderness. This is, I think, the only happy memory I have on that ward: lying in that bed, waiting for a blood transfusion, watching each twin move blindly towards the other, until they were both facing each other, their eyes shut, nudging their foreheads closer and closer until they touched. One opened his hand slowly, fanning the air with his fingers, and the other copied this gesture exactly. It seemed to me, then, that they had choreographed a dance, together in the womb, which they were now enacting before us: a performance of perfect unity. Then, as suddenly as it had started, the movement stopped. They slept deeply, curled around each other, comforted by the return of a familiar beating heart. When the twins found each other again, after a period of painful absence, the peacefulness I witnessed, the profound stillness in that singular encounter, the goodness and the power, this I will never forget for the rest of my life.

As I watched Kasi race round our apartment, assessing the damage, I saw another kind of love, equally powerful. She was taking in the mountains of laundry, the piles of dishes in the sink, the hospital-grade pump machine, the steriliser stuffed with bottles, my new, bulbous body.

'Do you have help, right now, with them?' she asked, shocked by the sheer volume of Babygros.

'No,' I said.

'It's just you and them?'

'Most of the time,' I said, then: 'I often get visits from my mother-in-law. And a friend of hers comes from the church.'

Kasi marched to the kitchen, rolled up her sleeves and started cleaning. She put the kettle on to boil.

'Where's Callum?'

'At work,' I explained. He only had two weeks' paternity leave as a freelancer.

'Okay, sit down.' Kasi slid forward two steaming cups of tea. 'Before the babies wake up: what happened to you?'

'Nothing happened,' I said.

'What do you mean, nothing happened?'

My memory was foggy: distant and confused.

Why did she want to talk about that?

'I had an infection,' I said.

'Why?' she asked.

I felt confused. I told her I couldn't remember.

Kasi found any lack of precision extremely irritating so she pushed harder. 'But surely you have your birth notes?'

'No,' I said. I explained that the maternity ward at my birth hospital operated on a paper-based system. Throughout the twins' pregnancy I had a thick orange pregnancy folder – stuffed with ultrasound scans and growth charts – but after birth the midwives took this away and in its place handed me three pieces of paper, stapled in one corner. These were my hospital discharge notes – and I was meant to present them as evidence whenever I encountered a health professional postpartum. I showed them to Kasi.

'Look,' I said.

She looked.

'These notes,' Kasi said, 'they read like they are half yours and half someone else's. Like they belong to two different women. To two different births.'

Does it matter?

'Yes,' Kasi retorted. 'It does matter. A lot, actually.' She began to pace around the room. 'How many other people does this happen to?' With Silicon Valley horror, she concluded: 'Frankly, this seems pretty messed up to me. All your information should have been digitised. Someone should be dealing with this in government. There should be apps, transparency, databases.'

I replied, meekly, that while I often found dealing with the NHS Kafka-esque, I was grateful to the welfare state.

The babies woke, screaming, and I lifted up my shirt, snapped a pillow in place under my nipples and began a strange shifting operation. I popped a baby under each breast, holding them in place like American footballs and settled in to feed. Kasi gasped as my littlest twin, Baby B, dwarfed by my prodigious breast, struggled with an explosion of milk.

'Your life is insane,' she announced, remarking on the squeaking sounds my sons made as they drank: 'Is that normal?'

'They have a floppy larynx,' I replied.

Kasi continued to stare.

'Nobody tells you,' she proclaimed, with great frustration, 'the truth about anything related to motherhood.'

It was a scandal.

The last time Kasi had seen me, half-naked, breasts out, had been on my wedding day, slipping into a thin silk dress. From this point on, my body had changed beyond recognition. With her customary attention to detail (intent, I think, on avoiding the same fate when she had children), Kasi wanted to know *precisely* how this had happened. How had I developed this magnificent potbelly, with its strafe-marks and scars? She politely called it my 'cushion': a gargantuan mass that flopped down over my pubic bone and jiggled like set jelly. In my numb state, I found her curiosity cathartic: I didn't have the energy to feel bruised or humiliated. As a male doctor wryly observed at my GP practice, examining the healing sutures in my vagina, there was not much dignity left to hold on to. I reassured Kasi that unless she had twins, this fate was unlikely to happen to her. But she wanted details. I explained that six weeks after my miscarriage, when I found out I was carrying twins, I had read an American book that said it was important to gain fifty to sixty pounds over the course of a twin pregnancy to give the babies a fighting chance if they came early.

'Huh,' she said. 'Really?'

'Oh, yes. Absolutely.'

Kasi raised an eyebrow.

Perhaps I had taken this to an extreme?

With the conviction of a zealot, I followed the diet laid out in the book to the letter. But my twins did not come early, and as I ate, I grew and grew and grew. On the day I gave birth, I weighed fifteen stone and my stomach bore no relationship to any belly I had seen before. In a lifetime of watching my mother carry seven children, nothing matched this. At thirty-four weeks, my fundal height (the distance between a pregnant woman's pubic bone to the top of her uterus) measured 45 centimetres. By thirty-eight weeks – and the last day of my pregnancy – my stomach had stretched into something grotesque and alien. The skin on my belly was so thin that you could see the boys' spines, and the moving lumps of their skulls and fingers and toes. Whenever they wriggled or kicked, their elbows and knees writhed at the surface – they were like puppies, racing around each other, or, at times, I thought: like an octopus. At first I enjoyed being so deliciously close to my children – I could watch as they responded when I spoke – but this soon transitioned to a deeper personal anxiety. As the pregnancy progressed, I felt increasingly at risk of ripping open. Two weeks before birth, an evil rash erupted on my belly. This was a blistering inferno – not unlike the rash that had appeared in my ear two decades earlier – that left pockmarks and scars. My belly burned and bled and it became almost impossible to walk. I wore a brace to support my children, and curved forward, wilting under the weight, a limping donkey. As I huffed painstakingly across my neighbourhood, in the days before I gave birth, strangers stopped me in the street, running to my side. 'Miss! Miss!' a group of teenage boys cried out, coming home from school. 'Do you need an ambulance?'

'No,' I wheezed, as they took me to the nearest bench.

'Do you think they might be identical?' I asked Kasi now, changing the subject. I had been told throughout my

61

pregnancy that my sons were fraternal – meaning two eggs, two sperm, two completely different genetic entities. For those who aren't familiar with the complexity of multiple gestations, the acronym on my file was always DCDA – *dichorionic diamniotic*. In layman's terms, this refers to having two placentas and two gestational sacs: two completely different pregnancies, inhabiting the same body. Internalising this information from the start, I had constructed a picture of the future that involved giving birth to two completely different boys – perhaps one fair like me, one dark like Callum – that sort of thing. But this did not seem to be the case. Yes, it was true that in terms of weight one baby was much smaller than the other, but they had, I pointed out to Kasi, the same mouth, the same nose, the same rolls of fat on their legs, the same creases in their skin when they cried. These similarities were now a cause of anxiety. When the twins were seven months old, I eventually swabbed the boys' cheeks with cotton buds and sent samples of their DNA to a lab at Norwich University. The results returned by post. I ripped open the envelope and found an answer. As I ran my eyes down two identical, neatly printed chains of DNA, I felt a sudden rush of relief. *Scientia potentia est.* Knowledge is power. Our boys were monozygotic twins – meaning that they were identical: they sprang from the same egg. Even in my fog of confusion, I had not been wrong, as a mother, to question the nature of their origin. But I did not know this then. And so I asked Kasi what she thought, and what others thought, doubting my own intuition.

'Yeah,' Kasi said, examining my twins. 'I think they probably are identical.'

She turned her gaze on me. 'Why aren't your parents around?'

A loaded question.

'They're dealing with a lot, Kasi,' I replied, in a detached, pathetic sort of way. 'Their house burned down.'

I revealed, then, that my father was going through a cancer diagnosis.

'They have to be in California for the biopsies. Besides, it's fine. I'm fine.'

'Is it fine?' Kasi retorted. 'Are you, though?'

Throughout Kasi's visit, it became clear to me that *it* was not fine. *I* was not fine. I did not think rationally, as I once used to. Confronting Kasi's questions was the first time I acknowledged, privately, that the nurse in the mint-green room might have been right: that I was traumatised. In that state of trauma, the sense of isolation was both debilitating and all-encompassing. It did not matter – empirically – that I was not *literally* alone, not ever, barring a few days in hospital, that first year of motherhood. It did not matter that I spent my first weekend recovering from a life-threatening infection, in the company of a dear friend who had crossed the world in my hour of need. It did not matter that having left hospital, I had been reunited with my husband and children. Alone? I was never alone. My children were always with me: at my breast, or strapped to my body, or asleep in the cots beside me.

When Kasi left, at the end of a five-day visit, other friends came in her place. My mother-in-law, who was a saint, visited daily, for hours at a time, her local church provided meals every evening for a month, my family supported us financially, and Callum parented whenever he could – changing nappies, washing bottles, helping me feed the babies throughout the night, despite the fact that he was commuting daily to a studio lot. Many, many people are far more alone in their parenting than I was – and yet this particular facet of depression, the sensation of being numb in the company of others, gave rise to an insidious, omnipresent solitude. In my memories of this period, I am *always alone*. It is difficult to recall anything other than an absolute sense of isolation, of standing naked in the psychological cold, unsure of where I was going, or what I had become – coupled with the firm belief that nobody else could understand or help me. This solitude was, in fact, the clearest indicator of the elemental force that now loomed above me, like a guillotine, shutting off contact with the world. In this altered reality, which only I could see, I was a lone woman battling a primordial menace, a monster of my own imagining, a new and constant shadow: the invincible spectre of loss. Faced with a sudden awareness that everything I loved could be robbed from me in a split-second, I struggled with what one might call final destination syndrome. If we were all going to die, imminently, and we were, what point was there in mothering in the first place?

Kasi wanted none of this. As she tidied and organised, she gave me instructions to follow: you must cook bone broth, and eat fermented food to build back the bacteria in your gut; you must sleep when the babies sleep, and if you cannot sleep you must hire a maternity nurse, she said, watching me take my pills, starting now, this evening, for a night, and you must do this until you get better. If you cannot afford a maternity nurse, you must ask for help from family members, and friends, to come and look after the babies, so that you can sleep and begin to recover. 'You are sick,' she said. 'You are not well.' She ran the numbers, with American brazenness, and told me exactly what we could manage. When I resisted, she stopped me and said, bluntly: 'Jess, this is important. You need to do this, for your mental health, for your body.'

That's how Kasi went on the attack.

'Have you guys been for a walk yet?' she asked the next morning over coffee, gesturing at our buggy.

'No,' I said.

'Why not?'

'I don't feel like it.'

'It looks pretty clean,' she said. 'You use it much?'

I shook my head.

It was a Saturday. Callum glanced at us, worried.

Since coming home from hospital, I had refused all requests to go out, insisting that it was safer to stay indoors.

'The sun is shining,' Kasi said. 'It's a nice day.'

'I haven't gone to the park since February,' I said darkly, as if this settled the matter.

It was now the middle of April.

'Callum,' Kasi turned to him, 'do you want to go to the park?'

'Yes,' he said, betraying me.

She got up from the table.

'Jess, I'll get your coat. You can hold my arm. If you don't feel well, Callum can push the buggy.'

In a flash, we were out.

I got to the end of the block and panic set in. The world was just as dangerous as I had imagined: everything was overwhelming. The wind was blowing. Branches were rustling in the trees; a plane was flying – too low overhead – it was falling out of the sky. A bus zoomed by and my legs began to shake.

'Are they breathing?' I asked Callum, who was pushing the buggy.

'Yes,' he said, 'they're breathing.'

'Are they breathing?' I asked again.

It was compulsive: I couldn't stop myself.

'Are they breathing?'

'Jess,' Kasi said, 'the babies are fine. They are sleeping.'

But what if they rolled up against the edges of the pram and suffocated?

'That will not happen,' Kasi said and took my arm, gently guiding me forward.

Before she left, Kasi did three loads of laundry, folding the family's clothes into neat piles on our bed. I came in while the babies were napping and helped her. We spoke quietly, as old friends do, and I asked how I could ever repay her. 'Consider it banked for the future,' she said. 'One day you'll get a call, and I'll need you, and you can be there for me then.' I promised that I would. I asked her then if she was worried about the babies. She leaned in and touched me, or at least I think she touched me, I have a memory of her touching my hand, and she said: 'I'm not worried about the babies, Jess. I'm worried that we're in danger of losing you.'

Trotula (or perhaps Trota) of Salerno, a twelfth-century female doctor of dubious origins (as much a medieval construct as anything else), documented what is perhaps the first European account of postpartum depression in her *Book on the Conditions of Women.* Echoing the Hippocratic authors, Trotula warned midwives that 'the brain suffers together with the womb,' and that 'the sign of this [suffering] is mental distress' in the woman. If the womb produced too much blood, after birth, the mother's brain was filled with water, and the moisture 'flowing to the eyes, forced them involuntarily' to shed tears.

I, curiously, did not shed tears.

In the darkened hush of my husband's sleeping, I looked through the netting of my babies' cots.

The stigma of mental illness in motherhood, as I experienced it, is real. As soon as people smell it on you, they pull away, as if your struggles were catching, like the flu. Out in the world, pushing my tiny babies in their wide double pram through sleety London streets, I would attempt to tell my story and watch others shy away. I learned to fall silent as other women aired their private grievances – inductions that lasted seventy-two hours and ended with a forceps delivery, or an unwanted emergency caesarean, or an umbilical cord wrapped around a baby's neck, or the awful snipping of flesh in a tongue-tied mouth or simply the endless sleepless nights, over and over again, unrelenting. I felt (rightly or wrongly) that what had happened to me was too frightening – that I had come too close to the impenetrable veil of death, from which there is no turning back. I knew, also, that there were worse stories, grief that dwarfed my own. A colleague of my father's had lost a baby full term just days after our twins were born. A stranger I met in the park spoke of her baby's visits to Great Ormond Street Hospital for Children, for treatment for cancer, receiving chemotherapy. I gave her my number, asking her to text me whenever she wanted someone to speak to, but she never did. She had shared more than she had wanted to share, and withdrew, overwhelmed, I think, worried that she might unravel. I listened, also, with unkind scepticism, to tales of the orgasmic home births in inflatable water pools, to a four-hour meditative labour in a birth centre managed expertly by a doula, thinking: *But what of nearly dying? What then?*

In the lonely, wordless days of my own depression, I grew increasingly estranged from the parents I saw around me: the yummy mummies in spandex jogging their buggies around frosted parks; the Instagram influencers, transforming their smiling infants into advertising platforms; the sling-wearing earth goddesses who would breastfeed for ever; the single parents with dynamic careers and strikingly intelligent older children; the stay-at-home dads and beautiful same-sex couples holding hands, as they perambulated proudly with their toddlers; the families who had used a surrogate or fostered; the high-powered bankers signing their offspring up to nursery at once; the wine-o'clock women, content with everything. How could I tell them of the mint-green room at the hospital in North London? Of the place I had entered, after my babies were born, of how close I had come to death? How could I tell them of the support I needed, mentally and physically, to survive, when I had not even been able to admit this to my husband, to my dearest friends? I was jealous of my peers who were not saddened by birth. I admired them, desired to be like them. In darker moods, I wanted to interrupt their happiness with troubling things. I wanted to ask: What secrets do you keep, that you too are not willing to share? What memories come to you in the night? How have you managed to survive? But one is not meant to ask these things of mothers. No amount of hypnobirthing or mindfulness or pre-natal yoga would have prepared me for these questions, which now burned constantly at the forefront of my mind.

Seeking answers, I gathered fragments.

Exhibit A:

The Gaki Zoshi, or *Scroll of the Hungry Ghosts*, dating from the twelfth century, housed in the Tokyo National Museum, (image no. C0016935, item A-1047). A hand-painted scroll from Heian Japan featuring a childbirth scene, in which a *gaki*, or hungry ghost, can be seen crouching beside the mother, waiting to devour the newborn child, prone in a smear of blood. Midwives, encircling the mother, do not notice the malevolent spirit, but in the adjacent room, somebody else does: a *miko*, or female medium, profile obscured by dark hair, hunches over a box of magic implements. Using the tools of her trade, the *miko* meets – and manages – the spirit perched beside mother and child, embodying its presence in the room. In twelfth-century Japan, birth was considered a door through which dangerous spirits walked. If a mother exhibited symptoms of postnatal depression, or psychosis, or physical illness, hungry ghosts were attributed as a source of her disturbance, and exorcists were called to attendance.

Exhibit B:

1628. Oxford. *The Anatomy of Melancholy.* When the famed seventeenth-century English scholar Robert Burton touched briefly on the nature of women's postnatal sorrow in his treatise on depression, he observed that his most troubled female subjects (his research pool comprised of 'nuns, and more ancient maids, and some barren women' and those that 'lie in child-bed *ob suppressam purgationem*') were wont to:

Complain many times [. . .] of a great pain in their heads, about their hearts and hypochondries, and so likewise in their breasts, which are often sore; sometimes ready to swoon, their faces are inflamed and red, they are dry, thirsty, suddenly hot, much troubled with wind, cannot sleep, etc. And from hence proceed, *ferina deliramenta*, a brutish kind of dotage, troublesome sleep, terrible dreams in the night, *subrusticus pudor, et verecundia ignava*, a foolish kind of bashfulness to some, perverse conceits and opinions, dejection of mind, much discontent, preposterous judgement. They are apt to loathe, dislike, disdain, to be weary of every object, etc., each thing almost is tedious to them, they pine away, void of counsel, apt to weep and tremble, timorous, fearful, sad, and out of all hope of better fortunes. They take delight in nothing for the time, but love to be alone and solitary, though that do them more harm: and thus they are affected so long as this vapour lasteth.

Such women were vulnerable to what Burton termed *'angorem animi,* a vexation of the mind'.

'Many of them cannot tell how to express themselves in words,' Burton complained in 1628, 'or how it holds them, what ails them; you cannot understand them, or well tell what to make of their sayings; so far gone, sometimes, so stupefied and distracted, they think themselves bewitched, they are in despair.'

Exhibit C:

1831. An article titled 'Observations on Puerperal Mania', published in *The New York Medical Journal* 1 and 2, suggests classifying cases of postpartum depression around severity of symptoms. Treatment, however, remains uniform: tepid baths – between 94 and 97 degrees – and a steady course of opium.

Exhibit D:

1858. Paris. *Treatise on Insanity in Pregnant, Postpartum and Lactating Women.* Working at the women's asylum of Salpêtrière, Dr Louis-Victor Marcé methodically categorised 310 cases of postpartum depression and psychosis in women. Drawing on the Hippocratic corpus, Marcé hypothesised, like the Greeks before him, that postpartum depression was caused by subtle, somatic changes in the body governed by the womb. He was among the first to identify and differentiate clinical aspects of specific syndromes which he considered unique to pregnancy, arguing that maternal insanity, while sharing characteristics with other mental health disorders, merited a classification of its own as an autonomous form of psychoneurotic disturbance unique to mothers.

Exhibit E:

15 July 1885. Letter to Martha Allen Luther Lane, from Charlotte Perkins Gilman, author of *The Yellow Wall Paper*, following the birth of her child:

> *... I feel as though I were drifting open eyed into insanity ... What seems most suspicious to me is that I no longer care much about whether I live or die, do much or little, cause pain or pleasure ...*

Exhibit F:

'Do publish those letters,' Virginia Woolf urged her friend Margaret Llewellyn Davies, pacifist, and General Secretary of the Co-operative Women's Guild from 1889 to 1921, 'they are so amazing.' Responding to Woolf's encouragement, in 1915 Davies published 160 letters, written by working-class mothers, all members of the Co-Operative Women's Guild. The testimony was explosive. 'The notion that pain and motherhood are inevitably connected,' Davies wrote in her introduction to *Maternity: Letters from Working Women*, 'has become so fixed that the world is shocked if a woman does not consider the pain as much a privilege as the motherhood.'

Letter 12, anonymous: 'I Dragged About in Misery'
It is lack of knowledge that often brings unnecessary suffering.
    Wages 2£ 2 shillings. Eight children, one still-born, four miscarriages

Letter 16, anonymous: 'A Nightmare Yet'
... the baby was a fine, healthy boy weighing over 12 pounds. Bad as was the effect on my bodily health, the mental effect was worse. I nearly lost hope and faith in everyone. I felt that even the baby could not make up for the terrible strain I had undergone ...
    Wages 25 shillings, three children.

Letter 20, anonymous: 'Stead's Penny Poets'
A miscarriage followed in consequence of the strain ... the physical pain ... threatened me with madness, I dare not tell a soul. I dare not even face it for some time, and then I knew I must fight this battle or go under ... You may say mine is an isolated case. It is not.

Wages: 32 shillings to 40 shillings: Five Children, one miscarriage.

Letter 136, anonymous: 'I wonder how I lived'
I do hope you will not feel that this letter is morbid, and that I delight in writing horrors, for I do not ... when I look back to my early married life I could cry for the girl who endured so much for life that was wasted ... please do not think I am miserable, for I am not, for I believe – in fact, I know – that there is a brighter day dawning for the mother and child of the future.

Wages 21 shillings to 30 shillings: four children, three stillbirths, one miscarriage.

Exhibit G:

1994. *Diagnostic and Statistical Manual of Mental Disorders IV.* Depression in the postpartum period is included as a modifier to major depression, bipolar disorder and other psychiatric illnesses.

Exhibit H:

2001. Melanie Stokes, Black woman, Chicago resident, and mother to a beloved three-month-old daughter, falls to her death from a hotel-room window after battling postpartum psychosis and depression. Following her death, Melanie's mother, Carol Blocker, commits her life to advocating for maternal mental health, demanding further research, funding and awareness for postpartum depression.

In 2010, the Melanie Blocker Stokes MOTHERS Act becomes law.

Exhibit I:

2018. *Mothers*, Jacqueline Rose:

Perhaps what goes by the name of 'postnatal depression' is a way of registering griefs past, present and to come, an affront to the ideal not least because of the unbearable weight of historical memory and/or prescience it carries.

I was not sure where to place myself on this continuum.

Increasingly, there were places inside me. Places I did not like to go to. Now, surreally, they returned, unbidden, in the form of dreamlike memories, memories that came when I was still. Standing over the sink washing dishes. Drying my hair with a towel. Hanging the babies' laundry on the line. Here the past becomes the present, and it is almost always dusk, and I am often barefoot walking up a dirt road. Somewhere in the distance, a song is playing, an American classic of the 1950s. I am careful where my feet are landing, avoiding the carcass of a toad, flattened by a car. There is another fragment, less commonly recalled, in which I disembark in a swamp of mangroves, and I turn, wearing a heavy pack, and watch a boat pull away into endless jungle. The worst comes after dark, when my children have gone to bed, and I am alone, fighting the infection in my womb, taking my metallic-tasting pills, waiting for my husband to come home. My children will be sleeping, and I will be making dinner in the kitchen, and look up at the windows, and I will catch my reflection, and suddenly, *just so,* I am back. I am back before a sink and a mirror, standing naked under a corrugated tin roof, at the edge of a forest. In this memory, there is always a spider sleeping on the wall behind me, large and black, the size of my hand, and I see, with a start, that the contours of the spider's body echo the contours of the bruising on my throat, and after birth, in my kitchen, in my present reality, my hand will compulsively go to my throat, and I will check that I am breathing.

You are alive, I will tell myself. *You are alive. You are alive.* This, perhaps the most vivid encounter with the past, is the most awful precisely because it is the most non-negotiable, the most excoriating, the most true.

SPRING

I take my boys' chubby hands, and run through the secret
woods, at the far end of the playground, weaving through
trees, slipping through the mud, hoping to delight them into
exhaustion. 'Puddles!' the boys shout, and stomp in them,
gloriously. It rained the night before and now that it is over,
we enjoy the freshness together. The air is wonderfully
clean. As we play, the sky opens, effervescent, an endless,
otherworldly blue. The twins crane their heads and point.
'Airplane!' they shout in unison. How it pleases them. For
weeks, if not months, maybe more, we have looked up in this
place, and seen nothing but an unfertile grey but now, oh!
Spring is making herself known. The children hurtle through
the little wood, stumbling often, dirtying their knees, their
smiles wide. I roam quietly behind them, remarking on the
light, on the shadows, on the greening earth, until my toddlers reach a cherry tree, in partial bloom, and here they stop.
A tree, once bare, now budded open. My sons marvel at this,
standing side by side, heads bobbing slightly in curiosity.
'Flowers,' they say, sticking out their hands. They touch the
profusion of buds. Flowers sleeping. 'These are babies,' I tell
them, as we examine the cluster, before correcting myself:
'They are buds.'

TALKING CURE

In motherhood a woman exchanges her public significance for a range of private meanings, and like sounds outside a certain range they can be very difficult for other people to identify. If one listened with a different part of oneself, one would perhaps hear them.

Rachel Cusk

Six weeks after my babies were born, Gráinne arrived, fresh from California. Indomitable Gráinne, who has no time for what she calls *ostriching*: living with your head in the sand, a woman who was a professional problem solver. 'Show me the bubbas!' she cried as she bounded up the steps to our apartment, full of excitement, green eyes flashing, in a light summer dress, her pale skin dappled with freckles.

'Does he look yellow to you?' I asked, handing her my baby.

'You know what?' Gráinne said. 'He does.'

Holding my child, she rushed through the door into our apartment. She began popping open the buttons of his sleep-suit on the living-room sofa.

'Pull back the shutters,' she ordered.

I pulled back the shutters, holding Baby A.

She moved Baby B to a place where the natural light was strongest. She touched his naked skin gently, examining his chest with glossy fingernails.

'Hey, little chub chubs,' she murmured, 'nice to finally meet you.'

I remember remarking privately on Gráinne's nails, how pretty they were, varnished with clear shellac containing flecks of gold. I watched her eyes moving as she analysed every inch of his body, neatly, methodically.

She nodded quietly to herself, then: 'Put his brother beside him.'

I put Baby A beside Baby B on the sofa. We looked at the babies together.

'Definitely yellow,' Gráinne said. 'No question about that.'

She took a photo of Baby B with her phone. 'Let me send this to my mom.'

Gráinne's mum was a midwife in San Francisco. I had written to her when I went into pre-term labour, and she had replied, generously, with a series of long emails detailing the pros and cons of C-sections and natural birth for mothers of multiples, the specific complexities, in her experience, of twin deliveries, and how to prepare, mentally, for having babies in incubators. *Keep your tush in bed*, Gráinne's mum had effectively written. *Stay still.* And I had obeyed. Gráinne fastened the poppers back up on Baby B's sleepsuit. Bringing her face close to his, she rubbed his nose with her shellacked finger. He stared at her darkly, then kicked his legs.

'Don't worry, bub,' Gráinne said; 'my mum'll know what to do.'

Owing to the eight-hour time difference between London and San Francisco, the response came back from Gráinne's mother that afternoon, while we were out in the park with the babies.

'That's prolonged jaundice,' Gráinne's mum declared over Facetime. 'Go see a doctor. I don't think there's any crazy rush, but get him into the GP first thing tomorrow.'

Panic, on my part, immediately set in. I spoke rapidly to Gráinne. Gráinne listened. When I finished, she said: 'This is not your fault.' But it *was* my fault. In the weeks since Kasi had left, my condition had worsened dramatically. I saw death everywhere, everywhere, everywhere. In the buggy. In the cot. In the water. In the swaddle. In the bottles. On the air. Nothing was clean enough. Nothing was safe enough. Any second, any day or night, one of my babies might suddenly die.

So I asked, whomever I was with, which was mostly Callum, urgently, obsessively, every five minutes, to check on them.

'Are they breathing?' I would ask. Even when I was holding them. Even when I could see that they were breathing.

I refused to wear the babies in a sling, convinced they would suffocate against my body, and I would not notice, and I would look down, and they would be dead against my breast. I refused also to allow Callum to wear them in a sling, and when he disobeyed, marching out the door with a shouted: 'These babies need fresh air,' I became tyrannical, accusing him of vindictive acts of torture, shouting that he would murder our children, neglecting their needs, ignoring their cries, that some irreversible damage would befall our sons under their father's watch. And I was paradoxically angry that Callum was not there enough, that he did not help enough, that he had abandoned us in our time of need – not of his own accord, of course, but because of the demands of the society we lived in, which forced him from my side when I needed him most. To make matters worse, where I felt either nothing or terror in motherhood, Callum remained euphoric: fatherhood suited him, he was full of blossoming happiness, which built a gulf between us. Where I was empty, he was full, and where I was not empty, I was miserable. I criticised him constantly: the way he held the babies, his lack of care, his failings. I would not let him touch me or come near me and over time, out of necessity, he had begun to actively resist my neurosis. This cemented my conviction that he was an enemy: that he did not understand me, would never understand me. We argued. Finally, when I came to Callum asking if our son looked jaundiced, he urged me, angrily, not to worry. It was a trick of the light. So I asked his mother when we went to her house for tea that afternoon.

'Does he look yellow to you?'

'No,' she cooed at him, lifting him out of the pram. 'Of course not, he's caught the sun. Darling little boy.'

My mother-in-law gave Baby B a kiss on his tiny forehead and he gurgled happily.

And it was true, then: he did not look particularly yellow, but I was convinced.

So I asked.

Again.

And again.

And again.

'Please,' my husband said, 'stop. I promise you, he's fine.'

But was he fine? Baby B's colour continued changing overnight until the whites of his eyes were yellow and I knew what jaundice looked like.

Our twins had been severely jaundiced when we finally escaped the postnatal ward after our first week in hospital. Once we had arrived back in our home, we had four more days of what's called 'hospital from home' care, running a makeshift ward from our living room. My family and I owe a great debt to the welfare state – not once did we see a bill – instead, strangers came to our door to heal us. A Northern Irish nurse arrived first, direct from our local hospital, wheeling in two carry-on suitcases that sprang open to reveal innovative machines.

'What are those?' I asked.

'Biliblankets,' she replied, 'never done twins before.'

And she set about expertly to install them in our living room.

She explained, as she worked, that the twins were to sleep naked on these space-age blankets, which plugged into an outlet and were powered by a small motor that resembled a vacuum cleaner. We had to keep our children on the blankets all day and all night, wearing little felt eye-masks and hats.

We must only take them out to change nappies – and once finished, we must immediately pop them back inside these portable cocoons of light.

'All right?' she asked. 'Ready?'

We stripped down the twins to their nappies. She pricked their skin, squeezing droplets of blood from each of their heels. The babies screamed during this, and I soothed them, and then we laid them each down on the thick blanket, and tied them in place with cotton strips, so that they could not wriggle off the healing waves of light. Once the babies were strapped down, we swaddled them loosely in a blanket, adjusted their little sunglasses, and switched on the machines. The sleeping pods drenched our babies in bright UV light, to help their bodies heal. I breastfed them like this, stiff, sunglasses-sporting babies, incarcerated in UV light, glowing bright in my arms, each hooked to a machine that roared like a space heater. Callum put a clipboard at the end of each baby's cot on which he would record numbers of nappies and feed times, and precisely how long they had been out of the blankets. He and I took shifts sleeping on the sofa in the living room so that we could tend to them when they cried – and they cried quite often – understandably I think, given the situation. I did not feel well, but I continued to be active – bounding up and down the stairs, picking my babies up to feed, passing them to the nurse, hovering anxiously over them. I had left hospital on a diet of painkillers and iron supplements, while Callum administered a shot of anti-clotting agent into my thigh every evening to prevent pulmonary embolism. At home, the babies drank constantly, in tiny amounts, strapped in their biliblankets and I became a milk machine slumped in the shower, examining the unfamiliar terrain of a foreign body: breasts riddled with stretch marks, soul disembodied. I leaked constantly, and gave up wearing shirts indoors, so that I could hoist my space-age babies onto the pillow strapped round my waist and hold them in place to feed. I did not feel like I was mothering – or married – or recovering. I felt locked in an endless firefight, battling a burning house. Three times a day, different nurses would come to check the twins' bilirubin levels, squeezing blood from their heels as they screamed. My favourite remained the nurse I met on the first day, from Northern Ireland; she possessed a wicked sense of humour. Every time she entered our apartment she cracked a joke about the vampiric nature of her job. 'Sorry,' she'd say, 'it's me again.' She chastised the babies when their blood did not come easy – 'naughty boy' – and also soothed them when they cried: 'You'll be back with Mummy soon.' She also assured us they were fine, and I believed her. She repeated this mantra with a confidence I trusted. Of Baby B she said, 'He's small but he's not that small', telling me of the babies she tended in the NICU, all of whom were heartbreakingly tiny, and this endeared me to her. She made sure I knew where I was on the scale of mothers' suffering. My problems were in the category of: *Not serious. Soon Over. Don't Worry.* By the end of the third day, I had fallen in love with this woman: never once did I doubt her. I thought her heroic, steady, kind. With her help, the yellow saturation soon faded from the babies' skin. I was relieved when they got better, but sad to see the nurses go. What would I do in the absence of their kindness in my life? 'Please stay,' I said, as the woman from Northern Ireland packed up the blankets. But she could not stay: other babies were in need of her expert attention.

In the absence of the nurses, I grew frightened. I could not sleep when the babies slept, and I began behaving oddly. During my second hospitalisation, memories surged up: memories I could not control. I felt I had no words for the emptiness that afflicted me. I am numb, I said to Gráinne, and in my numbness, I feel nothing towards my children, I no longer know *who* I am, or *what* I am, or *how* I am meant to move forward. I am frightened that I will die, because of numbness, that I will not survive. I am frightened of the infection surging up, unbidden, that has no source. That will not go away. I am frightened that I will hurt myself, that I will hurt them. I think of Medea's bone-chilling pronouncement in Euripides: *I go to slay my children*. Lamia, the beautiful Libyan queen turned child-eating monster, cursed with insomnia. Of the German fable *Der Weiss Frau*. The Mexican fable *la Llorona*. I think of how, in both of these fables, a mother drowns herself and her children vengefully in a river, then haunts the water's edge, eternally lamenting. I do not question the misogyny woven through these stories, these parables of warning. Instead, I internalise the anxiety. The anxiety that if I articulate my own depression I will become them.

I confessed all this to Gráinne, in our kitchen, and Gráinne listened, cocking her head to one side.

'Have you told anyone else this?'

'No,' I said. She took an elastic band from her pocket, sweeping her hair into a messy bun. Gráinne is a natural redhead, but when she tied her hair up at the back, she revealed a punkish strip of hair, cut short at the nape of her neck, died hot pink.

'I don't think,' she said then, 'that your baby's jaundice is the only thing people around you aren't picking up on.'

Gráinne spoke then, directly.

She used the word *changed*, and she used the word *depression*, and she used the word *serious*, and these words, spoken with her signature clarity, with her clinical sharpness, scared me.

The medieval mystic and Englishwoman Margery Kempe (c. 1373) could not read or write, so when she recorded her life story in the form of a book, it was her son who wrote first, and then, it seems, a monk. In the amalgamate texts produced by Kempe and her amanuensis, the unnamed narrator refers to Kempe in the third person, always as *the creature*. As in:

> *When the creature was twenty years of age, or somewhat more, she was married to a worshipful burgess and was with child within a short time, as nature would have it. And after she had conceived, she was troubled with severe attacks of sickness until the child was born. And then, with the labour-pains she had in childbirth, and the sickness that had gone before, she despaired of her life, believing she might not live.*

Kempe was famous in the Middle Ages for prolific weeping. She wept at the cross. She wept in cathedrals. She wept in town squares. She wept at the pilgrimage sites of Europe. Everywhere she went, she wept, and everywhere she wept, she was asked, in her own language, Middle English: 'What eylith þe woman?' Or: 'What ails you, woman?'

It feels significant (to me at least) that Kempe's answer to this question, presented, boldly, in the format of a book, opens with a traumatic story of birth. Not Kempe's own emergence into this world but her experience of giving birth, her experience of coming into motherhood. For months after the difficult birth of her first child, plagued by what many scholars now consider postpartum psychosis, Kempe suffered visions, witnessing (or so it seemed to her):

devils opening their mouths all alight with burning flames of fire as if they would have swallowed her in, sometimes pawing at her, sometimes threatening her, sometimes pulling her and hauling her about, both night and day during the said time.

Kempe's behaviour towards her family changed: *She slandered her husband, her friends and her own self. She spoke many sharp and reproving words; she recognised no virtue nor goodness.* She became increasingly suicidal. She bit her own hand so hard, she carried the mark for the rest of her life. Relatively speaking, Kempe got lucky. Were it not, Kempe's amanuensis recounts, for the constant vigilance of the creature's friends, family, priest and deity, *she would have killed herself many a time,* as the spirits stirred her to do.

John Winthrop, Puritan Governor of the Massachusetts Bay Colony, recalled in his journal, *The History of New England, 1630–1649,* the curious case of Dorothy Talbye (not so lucky), hanged at Boston for the murder of her three-year-old daughter Difficulty. Before motherhood, Winthrop wrote, Dorothy had been a woman 'of good esteem for godliness'. But after the birth of her children, Dorothy (like Kempe) changed: 'falling at differences with her husband, through melancholy or spiritual delusions', Winthrop observed, 'she sometimes attempted to kill him, and her children, and herself by refusing meat'. For these infractions Dorothy had been severely disciplined: excommunicated by her congregation, bound and chained to a post, beaten and whipped by her husband. At trial, Dorothy remained for the most part mute. Finally, after a period of prolonged torture, she confessed to breaking the neck of her daughter to 'free it from future misery'. Governor Winthrop, horrified by the filicide, sentenced Dorothy to death in 1639.

On 20 June 2001 in Clear Lakes, Texas, Andrea Yates, suffering from postpartum psychosis and schizophrenia, drowned her five children in the bath, one by one. The eldest, Noah, was seven. The youngest, Mary, was six months old.

The fear that maternal filicide is associated with maternal madness is not unique to me. The spectres of Andrea Yates, Dorothy Talbye, Margery Kempe terrify me: they haunt the depths of what Adrienne Rich called *the maternal heart of darkness*. But those children, I think, and feel sick. I know, objectively, that where these women failed their children, society also failed them. But that does not stop me feeling frightened, when the symptoms of depression begin, of being classed as Medea, Medusa, Monster: as *one of them*. Of becoming *one of them*. Callum reads this and reassures me: 'But you never would have hurt them,' he says of the children. 'You never, ever hurt them, or spoke cruelly to them; I never worried about them in your company, you showed them so much tenderness, such love.'

'No,' I agreed, 'I would never have hurt them.' But as the symptoms of depression deepened, as my hysteria spread, I felt that if society (my friends, my family, colleagues, health professionals, strangers on the street) perceived me as an unhappy mother, they would perceive me as a monstrous mother. They would draw no lines of distinction between sadness in motherhood and violence in motherhood; they would conflate the two. And so I embarked on a great, pernicious lie. I hid my symptoms from Callum, his mother, my parents. I did not tell them the full extent of my thoughts, my fears, I expressed them only when I was alone, after the babies had gone to bed, the anguish, the silent rage. To be among them, as a new mother, the Andrea Yateses, the Dorothy Talbyes, the Margery Kempes. The disgust then, the abhorrence. The self-loathing. I should not have done this. Andrea Yates, Dorothy Talbye, Margery Kempe demanded attention, required support. They required understanding. So, too, their victims: their slaughtered and abandoned children. Why was it so shaming, so difficult for me, to stand beside them, as Adrienne Rich had stood beside Joanne Michulski, mother of eight, who murdered her two youngest children, on the front lawn of her suburban home in 1978?

I come back, as we must, to Joanne Michulski, Rich wrote in her controversial conclusion to *Of Woman Born.*

Desperation, surely, grew upon [Joanne] little by little. She loved, she tried to love, she screamed and was not heard, because there was nothing and no one in her surroundings who saw her plight as unnatural, as anything but the 'homemaker's' usual service to the home. She became a scapegoat, the one around whom the darkness of maternity is allowed to swirl – the invisible violence of the institution of motherhood, the guilt, the powerless responsibility for human lives, the judgments and condemnations, the fear of her own power, the guilt, the guilt, the guilt. [...] The scapegoat is also an escape-valve: through her the passions and the blind raging waters of a suppressed knowledge are permitted to churn their way so that they need not emerge in less extreme situations as lucid rebellion. Reading of the 'bad' mother's desperate response to an invisible assault on her being, 'good' mothers resolve to become better, more patient, and long-suffering, to cling more tightly to what passes for sanity. The scapegoat is different from the martyr: she cannot teach resistance or revolt. She represents a terrible temptation: to suffer uniquely, to assume that I, the individual woman, am the 'problem.'

Mothering through hysteria, I cast myself as scapegoat. I thought myself perverse, mutilated, corrupt. Unspeakable names bubbled up, unbidden, from some deep well of collective ire, fuelled by the stigma of the 'bad mother': it was not the task of mothering that was difficult, no, in my unhappiness, I was difficult. I was *the problem*. I had broken ranks. I had brought this on myself. To speak out was to be exposed in my badness, so *do not*, I thought, *do not speak out*. In doing so, I dampened my own rebellion. But silence would not cure my affliction.

In her book, *The Collected Schizophrenias*, Esmé Weijun Wang, herself 'afflicted' with shizoaffective disorder, rightly points out that the word 'afflict', in the terrain of mental health, carries its own 'neurotypical bias'. The implications of this bias are real. A little over a century ago, my Irish-American great-great-grandmother was incarcerated for life in a mental health facility in upstate New York, after suffering a psychotic breakdown following the death of her husband and the birth of a new baby. Her children were told that their mother had died of a fever, and were raised by their extended family as orphans.

Six months after the birth of her son, in 2017, on holiday with her in-laws in the States, the Korean-American author Catherine Cho watched in horror, in a hotel room, as her baby's face 'twisted into a demon's face, with a disfigured mouth and dancing eyes'. Before being admitted to a psychiatric ward, Cho witnessed a blinding light in the hotel room extinguish a looming darkness, then heard the disembodied voice of a deity. Gripped by hallucinations, Cho, like Kempe, sought refuge in prayer. As Cho prayed, she witnessed a transcendence of time in which she 'felt like I'd caught a glimpse of another dimension, of the void, of the truth, of possibility'. During her episodes of mania, Cho's experience of reality echoed 'those moments in dreams when you are not sure if you're awake or still sleeping, but in psychosis, no matter how many times you try, you do not wake up'. Fortunately, with the help of her husband and her psychiatric team, Cho recovered from stress-induced postpartum psychosis and the following onset of depression. Rebuilding the ruptured bonds with her son, she took control of her own narrative, returning to the notebook she had kept on the ward to produce *Inferno:* an incendiary, stigma-breaking memoir published in the spring of 2020. I am interested by the imprint of the past onto the terrain of Cho's motherhood. Writing her way through psychosis, Cho reveals that long before pregnancy, she had been a victim of domestic abuse. She describes her abuse as a poison stored deep within her body that emerges, like a curse, in motherhood:

There, I thought. There was the place of anger and pain. I wasn't able to escape it.

Natalia Ginzburg, mid-century Italian essayist and novelist, ruminating on the aftermath of war, observed that:

> Someone who has seen a house collapse knows only too clearly what frail things little vases of flowers and pictures and white walls are. He knows only too well what a house is made of. A house is made of bricks and mortar and can collapse. A house is not particularly solid. It can collapse from one moment to the next. Behind the peaceful little vases of flowers, behind the teapots and carpets and waxed floors is the other true face of a house – the hideous face of a house that has been reduced to rubble.

So too, perhaps, a victim of assault when it comes to the parameters of her own body in motherhood. Reading Cho's lyrical prose, I will turn to Audre Lorde's axiom that poetry 'is a vital necessity of our existence'. That 'poetry is the way we help give name to the nameless so it can be thought'.

Governing theory holds that postpartum depression sits at the heart of a spectrum of maternal psychiatric disorders. At opposite ends of the spectrum lie *baby blues,* often brushed aside with a cursory *it will pass* – a mild mood disorder affecting up to 85 per cent of mothers – and the rarer Medusa of maternity, *postpartum psychosis*, impacting only 1–2 mothers in 1,000.

'I am *coping*,' I told Gráinne, when she came to visit. 'I get out of bed. I take my medicine. I wash. I clean. I nurse my children.'

'But that does not mean you are *okay*,' Gráinne countered. 'That does not mean you do not *need* help.'

The morning of my babies' six-week check-up with their NHS health visitor, Gráinne paced in the kitchen, Baby A strapped to her chest, unloading the dishwasher. The health visitor sat next to me in the living room. 'Breastfeeding?' this woman asked, smiling. 'Yes,' I replied. 'Exclusively.' The health visitor liked this. She put a hand on my knee and soliloquised about the benefits of breastfeeding for babies. She asked me to strip my child so that he could be weighed. Naked, Baby B looked yellow. 'He is quite yellow,' the health visitor said. I told her we were taking him to the doctor that morning. She nodded approvingly, her glasses at the end of her nose, and then busied herself charting Baby B's growth in the red book, before looking up with a smile. 'Good work, Mum!' No one ever refers to you by name. 'Baby's gone up a centile!'

Baby B had lost 9 per cent of his birth weight in his first week outside the womb, and came home weighing four pounds twelve ounces. This put him in the .2th centile for growth nationwide, when most children sat between the 9th and the 99th. What did the .2th centile mean? 'Well, if you lined up a thousand babies in a row,' I remember one doctor telling me, explaining away this minuteness, 'your son would be the second smallest of the bunch.' Smaller than most, yes, but tenacious, large in spirit, and anyway, size was not an illness, it was a feature of personality, and I had soon relegated his minuteness to a non-worry. I did not particularly care that Baby B had finally gone up a centile, now weighing a little over six pounds. I cared that he was yellow. His colouring had worsened and I had stayed up late the night before, googling everything under the sun. An initial survey of the results was Not Good. The health visitor wanted to see the next baby. Gráinne came in from the kitchen, wearing Baby A in a sling.

'Tell her,' she ordered.

'Tell me what?' The health visitor looked up, startled by my friend's appearance.

'The truth,' Gráinne ordered sharply, lifting Baby A out of his sling.

'Oh sweetie,' the health visitor sighed when I'd finished, 'we need to sort you out.' She read out questions and I graded my answers on a scale that ranked aspects of my emotional life from excellent to terrible – using a number system from one to ten. The higher the final count, the worse the psychological situation. I answered her questions – which centred on my emotional state, my sense of anxiety, my relationship to my children, my vulnerability to suicidal thoughts. I, like many women surveyed, lied about suicidal thoughts. I thought if I told her I was having them, she'd institutionalise me and take my children away. Before she began, the health visitor had said she would come back again in two weeks and I would have to take the same survey. If I was doing better, excellent. If I had not improved, she would refer me for further help. When I finished the survey it was clear that I was not, to use the medical euphemism of choice, Doing Well. She referred me immediately, for postnatal depression, but warned that the wait for a therapist, through local services, could last up to three months.

After the health visitor left, Gráinne and I took my yellow son and his twin brother to the GP, who sent us to the paediatrics team at the hospital with the mint-green room in North London. I began to feel agitated. I did not like returning to hospital. When we got into the triage unit, I held Baby B down, with Baby A strapped to my chest, as the doctor pressed a tiny cannula into my tiny child's tiny vein. Baby B screamed, turning his face from the needle. My heart began to race. Fear exploded in my chest. As the doctor broke the skin of Baby B's minute fist, I felt a cannula going into my own wrist and pain as the vein blew out. I saw a yellow bruise ripple up my skin like a scar. Tears came to my eyes. I started. Baby B squirmed out of the doctor's reach, screaming. The tiny cannula dislodged, and with it, my child's blood. What was wrong with me? 'I can't,' I gasped to Gráinne. 'I can't do this.' Gráinne held my son down, stroking his cheek, and singing in his ear, as the doctor inserted his needle and I sat blankly in the chair provided for worried parents, holding my second sleeping child to my chest. Baby B's hand was wrapped in gauze as the doctor fixed his little cannula in place. 'Come over here,' Gráinne said. 'You need to hold him.' I slipped one sleeping baby out of my sling, and picked up the wounded other, as Gráinne sat beside me, in hospital, on the day of her return flight to California, and I was grateful to her, for our friendship. She had comforted my son when I could not and seen what others had not wished to see, and she had set in

116

motion the necessary stages of recovery, for both Baby B and me. She had appeared in our collective hour of need, much as Kasi had a few weeks earlier. I wanted to touch her, to make sure that she was real. She was real, I reassured myself, and she was here, in the hospital with me, holding my eldest baby against her chest, as if it was the most natural thing in the world. 'Stay,' I whispered to Gráinne. 'Please stay.' And I held her hand, and though she could not remain for ever, she stayed until the last possible minute. She did not judge me, did not criticise me, did not shame me. I sat, and closed my eyes on the wipe-clean bed on the triage unit and held Baby B tight, trying not to focus on the tiny cannula jutting out of his tiny hand. We had to wait, the doctor said, for the results of the blood tests, and so I did what I did best, I offered my child my breast and he drank, as Gráinne tucked my matted hair behind my ear.

'You can cry,' she said, mothering me. 'I promise. It's okay to cry.'

But mine was not the crying kind of sadness.

The numbness I suffered was private and opaque: a sheer, frozen land, flat and unremarkable, barring the occasional outcrop of anger.

Years later, writing this book during the pandemic, I called Gráinne in California, asking what it was like to have stepped over the threshold of our apartment to be presented with a jaundiced baby and a mother in crisis. She choked up on the phone. 'It was awful,' she said. 'You were holding this tiny, yellow baby, and you were both so sick, Jess, and so vulnerable, there was a quality of vacancy in you I did not understand. You had changed. There was something dead about your eyes. You could not register emotions. I found this very frightening. I did not want to tell you this, but I cried,' she said. 'I cried the whole way home.'

By the time the results of Baby B's blood work came back, Gráinne had left, to catch her flight back to California, and Callum was on his way to the hospital. Baby B did indeed have prolonged neo-natal jaundice, of the kind that worries medical professionals. He was lucky, the doctor said: this jaundice was not caused by liver disease and would not result in cerebral palsy. Baby B's body was simply struggling to process the bilirubin stored in the healing blood clot on his skull – his magnificent *double cephalohematoma,* the large egg-shaped mounds of dry blood caused by his haemorrhage at birth, courtesy of the ventouse. This healing process was turning his skin a bright, vibrant yellow. On the one hand this was good: it meant he did not need any immediate treatment. His jaundice would improve as the welts on his skull healed. 'But ...' the doctor said, 'when we ran the tests, a couple of other things came up. The first is that your son is anaemic. That's not too big a deal, and we can treat it directly. But the second is more unusual. Your son has a clotting disorder.' The doctor cleared his throat. 'In layman's terms,' he said, 'your son has something similar to mild haemophilia.' He rattled off words I did not understand, something about how a specific protein appeared to be missing from Baby B's blood and that his slowness to clot had worsened the haemorrhaging on his skull at birth – those massive, calcifying lumps of dried blood, the M-shaped mounds on his skull, that so upset me when I held his head in the bath – giving him jaundice.

The doctor ran his hand through a shock of curly hair. 'If you can stop yourself, I recommend not looking this up on the internet.' He paused. 'In the meantime, your son will need monitoring.' Baby B would have to come in for more tests – and more cannulas – and he was not to cut himself, or fall, not to be circumcised or have his tongue snipped in case of tongue-tie. In a gesture of sympathy, the paediatrician added: 'He's very young and babies are strange. Sometimes their blood gets better on its own.' The doctor explained, very kindly, that at our son's next appointment, a paediatrician would confirm a plan for Baby B's care and that they would not treat his blood until he was older. He reassured me that there was no better time to have a diagnosis like this, that something man-made called Factor had come on to the market, which made treating haemophilia much safer for new patients. 'It will start impacting you, most directly,' he said, 'when Baby B is learning to walk, but you will cross that bridge when you come to it.' And anyway: that was in the distant future. 'Your son,' he reassured me, 'is only six weeks old.' This was the beginning, not the end, of a new and uncharted medical journey. The paediatrics team at the children's hospital would get in touch for a follow-up appointment. We could now go home.

I told our families about Baby B with trepidation. I did not tell them about my referral for postnatal depression. I determined to get better on my own. A week after Baby B's diagnosis, I woke again, feverish, my sheets soaked in sweat. The infection returned in my uterus, so too the horse-pill antibiotics. My father called, then, from Los Angeles: 'What matters,' he said, 'is that you get help and you get help now.' He offered to foot the bill. Callum went to work each morning and I continued to manage my children on my own. Seven weeks postpartum, bedbound, too weak to pick up my children, I'd nurse them lying down, refusing to turn away from them, despite how badly I wanted to. At night, Callum would groggily hold them in place as they fed, and by day I would drape myself round my babies, or prop them up with pillows, placing a baby under each breast, and let them drink, while I stared into nothing.

Eight weeks after the birth of my children, a sonographer in an NHS hospital, hunting for the source of my recurrent infection, identified a chasm, about the size of my index finger, in my uterus. Perhaps a scar, she said. Perhaps an open wound. This, then, was the culprit: a fjord of bacteria, bubbling away inside me, hidden in the dark. The options, to her, were clear: I must be admitted, now, at once, and go back on to IV antibiotics and have a surgery to scrape out the infected lining of my uterus, which carried risks, she said, of sepsis – or failing that, a hysterectomy. 'We have to admit you,' she said. 'We have to admit you now.' The mounting terror, then, the old, electric fear, shooting through me, the winding pain, the blood sloughing out, the gripping and the tugging, the pulling and the falling. 'No,' I said. 'No.' Alone in the consulting room. No. Do not. Do not. Touch me. No. I will not. No. I am not. No. I must go home. No. I have children to feed. No. I have milk to pump. 'But you have to,' the doctor said. I did not *have* to do anything, I said. I refused, point-blank, to be readmitted. The next day, I was back in hospital, speaking with another sonographer and then another doctor, who expressed a concern that the dangers of operating on an infected uterus outweighed the benefits: my cervix had closed. The surgery carried a high risk of perforation, which in turn could lead to infertility, and the doctor encouraged me, instead, to take my pills, and go in for daily, and then weekly, blood work to make sure the infection markers came down.

Callum hired the maternity nurse to start the first day I was back in hospital, and help look after the babies, for five weeks, four days a week, and give me an opportunity to recover, at last, from birth, a costly expense that consumed the entirety of our savings, and required the additional financial and emotional support of our extended families. Privilege here, my abundant privilege, had a powerful hand to play: generational wealth protected us, insulated us. Still: childbirth did not come without material cost. As a result of the maternity nurse and my protracted illness, we would not be able to afford full-time childcare for the first years of our sons' lives. When the boys turned one, Callum's mother would step in, three mornings a week, to help me write my second novel, but it would not be enough. A friend of Callum's younger brother, an artist, who lived round the corner, would offer to help, then, in the late afternoons, and I would try to write, stealing an hour there, an hour here, working in the babies' naps, in the evenings, whenever they slept. I would try and I would fail. I would fail, again, to deliver a novel. I would lose my advance on a contract: not a writer at all, now, but a full-time mother in a single-salary household. Without my additional income from writing, we would find ourselves unable to pay the rent in London, and abandon our apartment, moving in first to house-sit an empty property after a bereavement in Callum's family, and then into his parents' home, during the second wave of the pandemic, where I would carve out the time to write, relying entirely on the labour of Callum's mother, as we cared alternately for my sons in morning and afternoon shifts. I share this, not to argue that I have suffered (in fact, I'd rather not argue that at all) but rather to make the point (if I am making any point) that my experience is not universal: it is defined by monumental fortune, the fortune of 'resilience', the fortune of 'recovery', the fortune of falling, and failing, without ever really falling or failing at all, in the true sense, the absolute sense, of which I have no real understanding. My ability to survive, to heal from illness, to write these words now, as my mother-in-law plays with my children in her garden, is not testament to my tenacity, or grit, but testament to my extraordinary privilege, which cannot be excused, and must, I think, be acknowledged.

In terms of disposition, the maternity nurse and I were not particularly well suited to one another. Of this nurse's previous clients, all mothers of multiples, I was, she told me, with some misgivings, the first who had delivered vaginally, and the second, ever, to breastfeed. I found it difficult, lying in bed, as another woman brought me my children to feed and whisked them away. I insisted on continuing to nurse the babies myself. She disliked this, worrying, whenever I returned from my visits to hospital, that my babies were small and undernourished, urging me to abandon breastfeeding and pick up bottle feeding instead, giving formula. 'They are too small,' she said, and she was right. 'They need to eat.' She insisted also that I swaddle the babies, firmer, better, that this would help them sleep, and I watched her wrap my infants tightly, bound in their muslins, and laid down like prisoners in their cots. I thought her rule-obsessed, an authority figure who looked down on my mollycoddling – 'This *feeding on demand*,' she said: 'it is absurd.' Callum, too, pushed me to behave. 'You're sick,' he admonished, which I was. He had taken that week to work from home, in case I needed to go into surgery, and he wanted me to get better. 'Please,' he said, 'do what she says.' What she says? *You must feed every three hours, on the dot.* Any earlier, or later, is expressly forbidden. The nurse advocated boot camp for babies. Routine, pacifiers, synced schedule, cry it out. Her pseudoscience around babies, a kind of animal husbandry, demanded strict adherence to an English code: follow her instructions and the babies would sleep through the night. I found it strange that the babies were expected to behave like characters from a period drama. They were to nurse at three-hourly intervals precisely: seven o'clock, ten o'clock, one o'clock, four o'clock, seven o'clock, with a 'dream feed' at eleven before the last adult standing went to bed – and within each of these three-hour intervals the babies were required to nap for ninety minutes. At the start of the cycle, one would breastfeed each baby, for three-quarters of an hour. Then one would lay them on their backs and entertain them, in a detached, utilitarian manner beneath a baby gym for another forty-five minutes. Once they had fed and played, on the dot of the ninety-minute mark, one would swaddle one's infants, briskly, without fuss, and lay them down to sleep with a pacifier. They were not to be touched again until the remaining hour and a half had elapsed, regardless of any cries of displeasure. Every three hours the same cycle of events must be followed without fail. Should the children weep or wail for their mother during the time in which they should be sleeping, one was to ignore them, or hold one's hands over their eyes until they succumbed to the situation and gave in.

I hated this, as soon as it started. 'The twins' – I protested, feverish, in bed – 'are only ten weeks old. Why do this to them?' Until this point, I had given them all I had, in the form of milk and contact with my body. We had established our own pattern, our own form of broken intimacy. Yes, it was wild, impulsive, erratic; yes, I continued to be seriously ill; but we were in dialogue with each other, my children and I, their mouths on my breast, my hands on their bodies. It meant something. My milk connected me to them: they drank what they needed, I made what they

126

required. Breastfeeding was a crucial part of my performance of motherhood, my force of will to look after them. I wanted them to feel nourished, to feel safe, to feel held, and I understood, instinctively, that breastfeeding was a vital tool. The nurse did not care about breastfeeding. Uninterrupted slumber, I discovered, was the holy grail of her enterprise. A large baby, a happy baby, a swaddled baby, she told me, slept; so the nurse taught me how to swaddle properly, how to squeeze my babies' feet when they cried and rub their noses and hold my hands over their eyes, to induce fatigue. She introduced our family to a controversial technique called *mixed feeding* and implemented that *dream feed*, a massive formula bottle at eleven p.m., which we gave to the boys while they were sleeping. This innovation, she claimed, would eventually *push* the babies through the night. During this feed, she encouraged me to rest, but I rebelled, pumping milk that I could give the next day in bottles. After every feed she showed me how to burp them, rubbing their backs in a methodical way that I emulated, and later incorporated into my own routine, long after she left our home. Throughout, I shadowed her like a dog, trying to learn her secret wisdom. But I could not follow everywhere: I was too sick to walk much outside, so she took the babies to the park in the buggy, and I would watch her, leaving with the twins, through the window. Retrospectively, I think she saved my life, but I found the severance of my connection with the babies overwhelming.

Despite our differences, I learned to appreciate the nurse in our midst. She worked a quiet magic. With her help, my health slowly improved and over time I grew fond of her. I admired her no-nonsense approach to infancy; the cups of instant coffee she brewed; the stories she told in her sardonic, northern accent; her fierce, hawkish eyes; her manifest distaste for her clients (myself included), and her quiet, hard-won confidence with babies: her genuine passion for her trade. She was good and determined and her life had been hard, much harder than my own. She talked and I listened, and I realised this was a woman of reason. Routine was her rock: it was how she brought order to chaos. Who was I to judge her methods, or the bottles of formula she advocated? What did it matter, really, in the end, what the babies were fed, so long as they were happy, so long as they thrived? I have since come to believe that newborns are mirrors. The way we touch them and treat them, the way we approach them and try to control them, tells us far more about our own inner lives, about our own secrets and insecurities and belief systems, than any adult likes to admit to another.

From a medical perspective, the arrival of the maternity nurse was objectively beneficial, much celebrated in family circles. By the end of the second week, the fever had broken and did not return. Since birth, for seventy days, I had taken the metallic-tasting pills. I did not, now, require surgery after all. I slept at times, five or six hours in a row. Soon, I ended my final course of oral antibiotics, and, in the third week, when I took the follow-up tests at the clinic, my blood work showed that my body had cleared the infection. By the end of the nurse's engagement, I began to feel better, to go outside. I took Baby B to a cranial osteopath to help with the calcified lumps on his skull, which remained pronounced and extreme, moulding the little crown of his head into a mountainous valley. I saw a specialist gynaecologist, who laid out a new plan of care. The maternity nurse left, hugging me as she said goodbye. 'Control,' she said, 'staying in control: that is the secret.'

Slowly, inside, my wounds had healed. As they healed, I began to dream. I dreamed of bleeding, my body porous, leaking, as from a sieve, hands inside me, a flood beneath me. I dreamed of mangled organs. Of placentas, ripped into pieces. Of blood thickening, measured in a plastic bag, slopping in clear bowls, pooling like water on the floor. I dreamed of the going and the coming back, of the women, holding my head, saying, 'Don't cry, don't cry, speak, speak, stay with us, stay with us', thinking, *This is it. I am gone now.* And then, being gone. Really, truly, being gone. Until they brought me back. Until those women brought me back. Until all these women brought me back. I woke from these dreams atomised, a thousand fragile pieces of a former self. Strange bodies. Sleeping beside me. *Do not touch me. Do not touch me. Do not touch me.* In the split second of waking, I did not recognise them: my husband, my children. *Breathe*, I told myself. *Just breathe. You are alive. You are alive. You are alive.*

The blankness, then. The vast, impenetrable fog.

'Thank you,' the NHS therapist said, after I'd filled in a diagnostic form, full of bubbles and boxes and *rank this feeling from one to ten*, and returned it to her. She scanned my answers quickly, flicking through pages, then looked up with round, doe-like eyes. 'Why have you come in to see me?'

I told the therapist, a clinical psychologist specialising in perinatal mental health and family well-being, that when I looked at my children I felt empty. That there were no so-called happy endorphins, no breastfeeding connections, no experiences of maternal euphoria, no hours spent gazing into the perfect, sleeping faces of my children. That I felt, in a word, nothing. I did not mention the dreams, worried she would think they were hallucinations. I confessed to her, instead, directly, that I refused to leave the house with my children unless absolutely necessary. That I obsessively sterilised and then re-sterilised and then re-sterilised baby bottles. As to my own hands, I had washed them so many times the skin was completely raw. 'My main daily concern,' I said to the therapist, 'when it comes to them' – gesturing at my infants – 'is that, at any moment, one of us will die.'

After I spoke, the therapist rattled a toy in the babies' faces.

'It's very normal,' she said.

'Normal?'

131

'The worries you are describing.'

The twins gurgled at her happily.

'The babies at least seem like they're doing well.'

Were they, though? How did she know? My therapist, who, for the sake of anonymity, I shall call Grace, explained that she practised a particular kind of compassion-focused therapy.

She would like to lend me a book, titled: *The Compassionate Mind Approach to Postnatal Depression* by Michelle Cree. Grace believed I might be suffering from something called birth trauma, alongside, or maybe instead of, postnatal depression. I learned from her that the experience of feeling depressed after birth was not at all unusual. One in ten mothers in the UK experience the mood disorder known as postnatal depression. Experiencing full PTSD after birth was, she reassured me, actually quite rare: Only 1–4 per cent of women, she said, suffered the full spectrum of post-traumatic stress disorder after birth, though up to 45 per cent of women reported when surveyed that they felt their birth experience had been traumatic or, to use the euphemism of choice, 'negative'. Grace said she thought I might be in that 1–4 per cent category of mothers who developed birth-induced PTSD.

'Did you think,' she asked, 'at any point during or after birth, that you or your children were going to die?'

I nodded.

Had this been difficult to talk about?

'Yes,' I said. 'It had.'

I confessed to Grace that ever since the babies were born, I had struggled to find meaningful terms to express my state of mind. That I had discovered an experience of motherhood for which there was a startling – even violent – lack of vocabulary. A place where there were no words. I told the therapist that my family home burned down three months before the twins were born and that my father was diagnosed with cancer the week of my sons' birth. That I'd failed, twice, to deliver a novel and that I'd haemorrhaged in childbirth for reasons I didn't understand and that I'd had recurrent uterine infections and that the babies had come home jaundiced and that B had a clotting disorder and that for the past four months – give or take – I had spent each and every day worried that I would die. That I would die, or that my children would die, or that my husband would die, and if they did not die, that they would leave me, I would lose everything that mattered. I told her that when I was not experiencing a flash of paranoid fear, I felt numb. That I oscillated daily between two acute states, which I called the Numbness and the Fear. That I struggled to connect with other people, believing that I was a Bad Mother, paralysed by the knowledge of what did not happen, but could have been: the fear of the worst extreme. I felt, like Betty Friedan long before me, that I grappled with *a problem without a name*. What words would the therapist give the maternal experience I had lived through? How would she articulate the suffering of my own heart, when there seemed to be no common parlance for it? No accepted mother tongue?

Grace thought for a while, looking at my children, before remarking that there were *no easy answers*.

Which annoyed me.

But she was pleased to see that I was communicating my feelings, and if I was willing to continue talking about my problems, which she felt were entirely reasonable, there was, in her opinion, no pressing need to prescribe medication.

'Unless, of course, you wanted that?' She looked at me directly. 'Perhaps it could help?' she said. 'Medication often helps.'

133

I'd taken oral antibiotics for ten weeks.
I was done with pills.
'No.' I shook my head. 'No.'

Grace prescribed, instead, a talking cure.

I left the little meeting room and the therapist and a young Australian doctor helped me carry the wide double pram back down three flights of stairs to the ground floor. There was no lift in the building so I held the top end of the buggy and watched the squirming, red faces of my children, squinting in confusion, turning their heads from the harsh medical lights above them. At the bottom of the third flight of stairs, we reached the entrance and the therapist patted me warmly on the back. 'See you next week,' she said, and disappeared behind swinging doors as the babies burst into tears. They raged against the pram, against the place, against the world, and confronted with their rage I experienced a sensation of drowning. As the twins roared their displeasure, they gave voice to a hidden misery, shared by both mother and children. I tried to feed them, there in the waiting room, under the burning gaze of other patients' eyes. I put them to my breast and they screamed. I took out the little bottles of my pumped milk and gave them each a silicon teat, but they rejected this too, batting the bottles away, wailing even louder. Oh! They hated everything! When I held them both in my arms they thrashed at my breasts with tiny fingers, tears streaming down their cheeks. What was this new hysteria? Were they frightened? Had they remembered the nurses who came to our house, three times a day, to pinch vials of blood from their toes? Did the identikit consultation room or the therapist's manner recall the examining rooms that had inflicted such horror on us at the beginning? What about the staircase? Or the doors? Had these triggered my children, flooding them with unwanted memories? I hated myself, then, even more. I was a terrible mother. A mother who had inflicted her own suffering on her children. Taking them to a place like this? How selfish. How disgusting. How weak, and puerile, and stupid. They both continued crying, both refusing to nurse. Soon, I found myself shaking. I had brought them back into suffering. I had unlocked some potent memory. Of incubators, of harsh white light. Or worse? I suddenly thought. Had they understood in some way, my confession? Were they now reflecting back at me the tears I could no longer cry? My own repressed despair?

Enough! I placed the babies in their buggy, drew the twin hoods down and walked into blazing sunshine. The weeping did not stop for what felt like hours – but in reality, ten minutes later, they were asleep. As I walked my children home, I promised myself that I would never, ever, go back to that therapist's office. I felt a surge of anger: it was this woman's job, surely, to explain exactly what was happening. To present me with a specific medical language with which I could categorise my melancholy and pain. Why this cruel absence of terminology? Why this unspeakable taboo? At work, even there, in the clinician's room? Look at us, all these women on the street, passing each other in silence? As I walked, I wanted to scream. She'd given me a book. *A book*, she says. *No easy answers,* she says. What a joke! I texted Callum, pushing the buggy uphill: *COMPLETE WASTE OF TIME!!* Callum called from the soundstage where his show was shooting: 'I promise you Jess,' he said. 'It is not a complete waste of time.'

To my surprise, Grace rang me that afternoon, to say that she'd looked up my address on the system, and had found a new location, one that didn't involve carrying the babies in the buggy up three flights of stairs. 'Perhaps the health centre around the corner from you might work better?' she said. 'The doors are wide. And there's an available room on the ground floor.' Moved by this unexpected gesture of generosity, I agreed.

Later that evening, I began, also, to read the book she had lent me: *The Compassionate Mind Approach to Postnatal Depression: Using Compassion Focused Therapy to Enhance Mood, Confidence and Bonding.* As I read, I felt increasingly upset. What I had thought was my own unique suffering was not uniquely mine at all. Why do health professionals and family members couch suffering in such infantile terms? Midwives who handed us leaflets on *baby blues?* Promising the sadness will go away in a matter of days? Or hushed whispers of *mother's trouble?* Why did these people not speak more freely of the wilderness of motherhood? The way it isolates you? The way it impacts your relationship to your children, to your spouse or partner or friends or family, to the world around you? And if you feel afflicted by birth, but have no language with which to speak of it, how and when are you meant to recover? I did not know it then, but this was the first step of a prolonged healing process. That in asking these questions, I had started to hit back at the vast, opaque muteness of my maternal confinement.

From late June of 2018 through the end of October of that same year, over a programme of fourteen sessions, accompanied by two tiny infants, I went weekly to a little room, in our local NHS trust, with faded chairs and battered toys. During this period, memories alone served me, and with the mutability of memory, an inevitable blurring occurred. There was a birth, and there were babies, and a period of great sickness, and medical emergencies and midwife appointments and follow-ups. But as my physical health improved, the precision allocated by hospital visits vanished, and in its stead, the numbness grew, and with it a fog, a forest of vagaries. Delineating the passage of days and weeks and months felt impossible. Now, when I return, clear eyed, to examine what happened there, that same fog descends, through which the therapist appears like Charon on the River Styx: I, the passenger, and she, the ferryman.

SPRING

*In the park, one of my sons bolts out of the little forest,
and speeds across the sandpit, vanishing into the middle
distance. I sweep up the nearest boy in my arms and bound
after his escaping brother, catching him as he hurtles towards
a precipitous ledge, yanking him back to safety. 'Please
remember to stay with Mummy,' I say crossly to him. 'It
scares Mummy when you run away.' And immediately I feel
bad. I want my sons to have a sense of freedom, difficult
for twins. Now that my sons are free-ranging, I cannot do
many of the things other mothers easily do with toddlers: I
cannot, for instance, take them to museums or galleries on
my own or let them play in playgrounds that have multiple
points of access. Not because I don't want to, but because,
quite frankly, they escape. Gates, for instance, are a kiss of
death. If there are two, my sons at once separate and speed
towards each gate, in opposite directions, partly, I think, for
the entertainment of watching their mother careen franti-
cally from one corner of the playground to the other, partly
for the sheer joy of liberation. Whenever we are in an open
space, like the playground, which is quite often, I have developed a technique of positioning myself equidistant between
them, turning my head like an umpire at a tennis match,*

muscles twitching – ready, at any moment, to spring into action.

To help with the dilemma of managing equally matched toddlers in the wild, I have spent the last year teaching my sons Makaton, a variant of British Sign Language designed for babies, which allows me to communicate with them at a distance. Come back! I will sign wildly across the playground, and if they see me, and feel inclined, the boys will stop and respond in sign and return. I can also ask questions, which they answer eagerly, carving out shapes in the air with their hands. We play games in our silent language – identifying animals, signing the colours of the rainbow, putting shapes to feelings – and my sons enjoy this, I'm sure of it, the puzzle of communication, the game of it. It is something I started doing when the twins were ten months old, and signing has helped me hugely, connecting me to them in this gestural, peaceful way.

THEORETICAL ISSUES

The task of calling things by their true names, of telling
the truth to the best of our abilities, of knowing how we
got here, of listening particularly to those who have been
silenced in the past, of seeing how the myriad stories fit
together and break apart, of using any privilege we may
have been handed to undo privilege or expand its scope
is each of our tasks. It's how we make the world.

Rebecca Solnit

In the beginning, I had the distinct impression that nothing happened. Each week, I went at an appointed hour, and pressed a buzzer at the entrance to a local health centre, and gave my name to a woman at a desk, who rang a number and asked me to wait in the waiting room with my buggy, until Grace appeared at the doors and beckoned me forward. As I pushed my children dutifully towards her, Grace would smile, and pivot lightly on her heels, and lead me towards a narrow room with a narrow window and a narrow desk full of narrow things. The therapist's lair was a strange, medical environment that smelled, rather unpleasantly, of disinfectant. The room – which was multi-purposed and communal – bore no trace of individual personality. It was clean, and utilitarian, and simple, the kind of place you go complaining of a common cold, and are sent home, without fuss, to rest. Grace would sit where a doctor presumably sat at other times of the day, and offer me the facing chair and apologise, almost ritually, for the aesthetic shortcomings of this place. I would smile out of habit, rather than out of feeling, and say it didn't matter, really, where we were and begin the practised, empty chatter I had developed as a means of hiding my agony. I would sit on the floor, shaking rattles at my children while my thoughts drifted above them. I had fifty minutes to fill – no more, no less.

'It is difficult,' I'd add, gesturing at the babies, 'for me to talk in front of them.' Grace encouraged me to try. In order to heal, she said, to really heal from birth, inside and out, I would have to confront the past. I would have to understand what had happened to me there. I would have to give it *a name*. Rewrite and relive each individual event in order to integrate my birth experience, to change the way it had been stored in my brain. My therapist likened it to reorganising an over-stuffed cupboard: the cupboard of doom we all have under the stairs. I would have to take everything out and sort it. Fold the winter clothes neatly. Hang the ironing board. Relocate my husband's tennis racket. Box the Christmas ornaments. Chuck the odd, unwanted shelving unit. I would have to exhume every lived experience, every shattered piece of the puzzle, and put it back together. I would have to do this in order to mother. In order to escape the sorrow and the madness, the numbness and the fear: the endless, empty park, through which I moved my buggy in quiet isolation.

Sometimes I said very little. Sometimes I said a great deal. Very often I did not know what to say because I was frightened. Should I explain, for instance, that yesterday, when I smelled my son's forehead, and ran my finger gently along his downy skull, I remembered with atrocious clarity the open wounds the forceps had left around his fontanel, and it appeared to me, briefly, as if his wounds were still there, and I had a terrible urge to drop him or push him violently away? *No, no*, I would think to myself, *this is too much.* So I would stare into the middle distance and say nothing as Grace reminded me gently that the time was my own, to use as I wished. 'To speak of your depression. Or perhaps your daily life? Or perhaps your lack of feeling?'

She'd ask me, then, if I had felt something – anything – that week.

'No,' I'd say. And then, the next time, 'Well. Maybe. A bit.'

The motif of the unkempt cupboard, which Grace used often to describe traumatic events, vexed me. 'My mind,' I said to her, 'is not a wardrobe: it is a vast, opaque maelstrom.' My problems don't have boundaries. Neat *beginning, middle, ends*. They are not *stackable, foldable, cleanable*. The things that I remember – the fragments that hurt me – are chaotic and inconclusive and elliptical: they are not piles of moth-eaten knitwear, made lovingly by distant relatives, which could easily be sorted and thrown away – Marie Kondo style – with a gleeful invocation of minimalism.

Rather than sorting through things, I'd relate the telephone call I'd received yesterday from the paediatrician who had been managing my son's care at the hospital. How the female doctor explained over the phone that the clotting factor in Baby B's blood had dropped to the normal range. 'He's fine,' she said, and I could hear the emotion in her voice. 'I'm discharging him today.' I asked how this was possible, and she said: as far as she was concerned, baby blood was mysterious. Sometimes, she said, with the instruments of modern science at our disposal, we know too much, and our findings worry us more than they should. His clotting disorder was likely created by placental problems in the womb. As he grew, and produced fresh blood cells, Baby B's clotting factor resolved itself naturally without medical intervention. This pleased Grace, who nodded and smiled, and asked, 'How does that make you feel?' To which I answered numbly, *fine,* feeding the child at my breast, and then, meekly, that when I heard *placental problems in the womb,* I blamed myself.

Throughout, Grace spoke rarely, if at all. She was a woman whose own life I would know nothing of, who sat, sphinx-like, at the boundary of the unknown, asking questions. Of her private affairs, I could guess very little. She was ageless and ringless and had a tendency to wear her dark hair loose, which ran past her shoulders, and had a great many pairs of black wide-legged, fashionable trousers, of the sort you see in magazines, and delicate leather sandals. When she walked, she was light on her feet, and had a habit of sway-ing, slightly, such that I wondered at times whether, in her childhood, she had been a dancer. Grace seemed acutely comfortable with silence. Occasionally she would offer a leading question, or make an observation, but for the most part, she sat quietly, listening, a picture of serenity.

I was not a picture of serenity. The things I felt free to speak about were mundane frustrations – such as the challenge of getting to therapy in the first place. Twelve vertiginous stone steps led down from apartment's front door. I could not put both babies in the buggy and get them down and up the stairs on my own. I was not strong enough to manage bouncing the buggy down. I tried once, and was rescued by a stranger in the street. If I wanted to go on a walk in the morning, I had to time it with Callum's leaving for work, so he could help me down, or exit with a visitor, a friend perhaps, who came to tea, but then: how to get back inside? I was an independent woman, and relying on others humiliated me. Stuck at the bottom of the steps, unable to reach my door, I would plaintively call my husband's mother or brother or father, who lived five minutes away, and ask if they could come and help me.

Callum's parents tolerated my complex need for independence with bonhomie. They watched, gently, from afar, worrying – about the stairs, and the door, and how I never went out, unless helped – and whenever I admitted the truth and said I needed help, they always came, lifting my buggy up the stairs, and in case they were out, and I felt utterly overwhelmed, they gave me a key so I could wheel the twins to their house and have a cup of tea while I waited for them to return. But sometimes, when no one was available, and my body was still recovering, I could not get in or out. I would pass entire days trapped like this.

My isolation made Callum anxious. 'How do we fix this?' he said. 'How do we make sure you can get outside on your own?' I said I didn't mind – the staying in, the being alone. Because it felt important for me to say *I don't mind*, even if it was, at times, impossible, to care for newborn twins, and maintain sanity. It was important for me to be *well enough,* after months of illness, to *do this on my own*.

Looking for a solution, I bought a bicycle lock for my buggy online, and after a few weeks of trial and error, I struck on a technique for exiting the apartment. I would meticulously pack my buggy bag the night before therapy, filling it with spare clothes and nappies and toys and medicine, and whatever other thing I might need in an emergency, and attach it to the back of the pram. Half an hour before therapy, I would place the twins on the floor in the corridor, making sure they couldn't touch each other, and leave them, squirming on their backs like stuck beetles while I took the buggy outside, bouncing it down the steps and locking it to the Victorian railing. Running inside the apartment, I'd strap my bigger twin, Baby A, into a single sling on my back. Then I would squat down, and lift up my little Baby B, holding him snugly in my arms. With both infants in place, on my body, I would walk out and gently lay Baby B down in the buggy, then unstrap Baby A from the sling on my back, and rest him in his own compartment. Then I would unclip the sling and stow it at the bottom of the buggy, before setting off, blearily, to see Grace at the health centre. Eventually I hit upon a better fix – a double sling – loading the babies in, one on my front, one on my back, which let me wear the twins as I bounced the empty double buggy down our vertiginous flight of steps.

If therapy had not been a short walk away, I doubt very much that I would have gone. None of the Tube stations in my neighbourhood have disabled access: there are no elevators to the station platforms. Buses, then, were my only option for getting around on my own, and buses terrified me – and besides, often several would go by before I could catch one. You cannot ride a London bus with a double buggy if there is already another single buggy on it. I did not own a car, and taxis terrified me as much as the buses did. Before starting therapy, I had developed a habit of not leaving the house unless absolutely necessary: going to a doctor's appointment, say, or being forced out for fresh air at the weekend by Callum, whose chipper well-meaning-ness I increasingly resented. This meant that therapy days were very often the only days in the week when I took the twins outdoors on my own, and when the session had finished, I would wander round a park near the health centre, in an over-stimulated daze, looking at the flowers while the twins slept. I'd pass pretty women breastfeeding on benches, and happy children playing on the swings, and I would believe myself to exist apart from them, fundamentally different.

Eventually, I learned to use the therapy outing to see other new mothers who met weekly at the pub for lunch. Many of the women spoke in hushed tones of difficulties with husbands and nursery placements and their phobias of postnatal depression, which, thankfully, hand to heart, they had evaded. Not once did I tell these women where I had been before their intimate lunches, petrified of exposing my melancholy. The women talked about milk, and formula, and weight loss, and diastasis recti and *mumfluencers* and exercise classes involving buggies. I did not find these things easy to talk about, and invariably left early, pushing my twins before me.

'These intrusive thoughts,' Grace asked, 'these intrusive memories ... How would you describe them?' I thought for a while, and said: 'Vivid.' And then: 'Real.' And then, with some embarrassment: 'I mean, I know they're not real. But they're ... Well, they're different to normal memories. I experience them, as if they were alive. As if things I remember were here in the present, here in the room, with me now. Happening to me right now.'

'How does this make you feel?' Grace asked.

'Frightened,' I said. And then: 'Empty.'

Then she nodded, quietly, to herself.

'And how often do you think these memories occur?'

'What do you mean?'

'Do they occur once a day? Once a week?'

'Once a day.'

Rounding down optimistically, I deftly switched subject. In reality, it was an almost constant loop. But I did not want her to think I was, to use the pejorative term, crazy. There were daily instances, for example, when I would feel a sudden tugging and a ripping and pulling in my belly, and have the awful sensation of my life force falling out of me. Each time, afflicted by these memories, I would grapple with an eerie conviction that I had died, and this life, which I was living, was an illusion, a dream state, from which I soon would wake, or exit, or vanish.

As the sessions progressed, Grace encouraged me to pay attention to the specific qualities of the memories that bothered me. 'What triggers them?' she asked. She wanted to know how long they lasted and what kind of situations set them off. Rather than push them away, as I usually did, I was to remain present in them, to allow them full expansion in my mind, to stop and observe the memories that came to me, and ask myself, each time, what, why, where, how? I was to notice what I was doing when unpleasant memories occurred, and, if I felt able, to keep track of them, in a sort of diary. If keeping track of them was too difficult, too forensic, too taxing, which it was (I did not write anything down for months), I could simply acknowledge the presence of the memory with compassion, and if I did this enough, over time, I might begin to engage therapeutically with the painful feelings the memories brought up.

This all sounded farcical to me, but I listened politely. Grace urged me to say to myself, at the onset of a recollection: *This memory makes me uncomfortable, but I acknowledge and welcome its presence in my life.* I could also practise verbalising my panic. I could, for instance, turn to whatever person I was with and simply tell them I was experiencing an unpleasant memory or a stress-inducing feeling.

There were techniques she suggested. Breath work. Keeping one's feet rooted on the floor. Pushing a pressure point on the hand. If I did this enough, I might find myself able to ground myself, during these episodes, and if I could ground myself, I might better inhabit the memories and resolve the pain they caused me. Feeling less pain, I might start to be able to articulate better the things that troubled me. I might recall concrete episodes of time – rather than fragmented images and feelings – and begin to transform the shards of dislocated memory into a narrative. Creating a narrative, Grace promised me, was therapeutically powerful. It might help reduce the negative impact of traumatic events. As I worked through memories, I was to focus on the specific minutiae of each traumatic experience. I understood this to be an act of mimesis: I was to note down sounds or smells or slivers of light that in turn led to a complete image and then a complete scene, and then a complete episode, which could, she suggested, be stowed away properly as a neat and ordered event – a decorative object in the kingdom of memory. She encouraged me to give voice to the specific memories of birth I found upsetting. 'When you see these things,' she would ask, 'the things that interrupt your thoughts, what do you see most often?'

'Blood,' I would say. 'My children's, my own.'

As I shared these things, Grace guided me towards a process of excavation that would, she warned me, initially feel extremely uncomfortable, but could be helpful in the long term. I should try my best to write down the details of any fragmented memories of birth, whenever they occurred to me. I did not feel able to write, so I decided to treat my investigation of the past as if it were a mind game, and I preferred to do this when the sun was shining. Sitting on the park bench, after my weekly session with Grace, I would start with the first thing that came to mind: something mundane, and seemingly insignificant. Perhaps the texture of the compression socks I wore in the mint-green room, to avoid blood clots? Yes. I would grab at this and then deliberately and painstakingly recall the exact quality of the tightly woven mesh, I would see its thick seam, and where the elastic in that seam bit uncomfortably into the fat beneath my knees. This uncomfortable biting sensation of the socks led me to think of the arrangement of my body in bed, and the gown I wore, and the little table to my side with the thin, white plastic cup and an uneaten apple given to me by the hospital and a small paper tray of pills. From the side table, I built outwards. My thoughts leapt in time, and I recovered an image of my hand, in which the blood had scabbed around a cannula in a vein on the back of my fist, and this in turn helped me remember that I had breastfed both babies, as I received a stranger's blood to replace my own, three days after my sons were born, and that I had cradled the bruised heads of tiny infants and thought, during the transfusion, looking at the bloody, dirty cannula in my hand, my hand with its peeling, blood-stained bandage and the blood-filled drip, I had thought then how strange it was that my milk was also made of blood and that this blood-milk aspect of mothering was not what I had wanted or imagined, and how that not-wanting-or-imagining made me unhappy. Milk in general, I told Grace, made me unhappy.

The hospital-grade electric pump, which my husband rented from a Swiss brand with distributors in the UK, arrived in the second week of our twins' lives, and took up a position of great importance on the far side of our kitchen table, beside the wall, where it could be easily plugged into the outlets below. The kitchen was a good location for pumping because the kettle was never out of reach, and the babies slept with us in our room so couldn't hear the noise. For those who have not pumped, it is an unfortunate business: I have yet to meet someone who has enjoyed their time at a milk station. Pumping is an unpleasant, uncomfortable pursuit not simply sonically, but physically. The pump consumes the breast, mechanically – yanking the nipple forward, while pummelling the glands in the areola in a suction pattern – there is a constant clenching and releasing, and if you are sensitive to such things, as I am, you feel stripped, oddly, of your essential being – over and over again – become, rather than a mother, a production line. The nipple swells inside the suction cup until it is about the size of a thumb, and emerges mangled. Sometimes this is painful. Sometimes not. Over a day of pumping and feeding, I passed hours like this: sullen, attached to a machine, wringing every last drop of liquid from my body. The milk emerged slowly, at first, without enthusiasm, but as the engine roared into life and the Swiss pumping became increasingly frenetic, the dam would break, and my breast would fill bottle after bottle. Over time I grew used to this milking, and tended to quietly evaporate, as soon as the pump turned on, and in this numb place, my thoughts would drift until my mind was empty, entirely emptied. And after emptiness? Exhaustion.

Death, danger, sickness, losses, all the ill
That on the children falls, the mothers feel,
Repeating with worse pangs, the pangs that bore
Them into life, and though some may have more
Of sweet and gentle mixture, some of worse,
Yet every mother's cup tastes of the curse.

Lucy Hutchinson, *Order and Disorder*, 1679

'I am so tired,' I announced to Grace that week, milk leaking through nursing pads, soaking my shirt. Too tired to do anything, to find space to breathe, to make myself a cup of tea, to brush my teeth, to shave my legs, too tired to adequately comfort my babies. They hated the utilitarian awkwardness of my double sling. They didn't want to be jostled, or shoved under their mother's breasts like footballs. If they slept on me, they wished to sleep alone, cocooned in blissful totality, without giving way to the needs of the other. With my twins, I lamented, I am always interrupting one's intimacy to help the other and this upsets them, for my babies crave intimacy – they want my singular attention. 'Because of this, they are never satisfied,' I said. 'I never seem to please them. I feel at times that I am their torturer,' I said to Grace, 'and they are my hostages.' I worried about this often: that my babies disliked me. That I disturbed them. That I was responsible, on some deep level, for their vast and inarticulate unhappiness.

Two of Callum's friends came for dinner. A young couple, childless, planning a year-long trip round the world. Next year, they said, they would travel to Greece, where they would work for several months supporting Syrian refugees. We took them to look at the babies while they were sleeping. My babies did not look like normal babies, they looked small and wizened and unhealthy, and I could see the shock on our friends' faces. They were anxious for us. They seemed, to me at least, to fear for our children's safety. Nearing the end of the meal, one of them asked a question: how did we feel, he asked, morally, about having babies in the context of climate change? Speaking from his own perspective, he believed that having children was a profoundly selfish act. Far better, he said, to die out, now, in this generation, than put additional strains on the planet by self-replicating. On ethical principles, he announced at the dinner table, he has decided not to have children. Childlessness appealed to him: he would rather remain an artist than become a father, and then he turned his attention on me – and asked me pointedly, as a woman who used to be an artist, and was now a beleaguered mother, what I thought of his radical stance on parenthood. 'Do you,' he asked, 'consider the act of creation selfish?'

I replied, equally provocative: motherhood is a profoundly selfish act. I did not ask my children whether or not they wanted to come into this world. I desired children, and so I had them. Motherhood is an experiment, the outcome of which we are never certain. I do not know when I make something whether it will be good or bad, whether it lives or dies. 'Many of the things I have made as a mother,' I said, 'lived for a while, and then died.'

That summer a woman came to my door. She ran a local charity supporting struggling mothers. It was the outset of Ramadan, and she came during her fast, wearing the most beautiful embroidered *abaya*. I told her I felt very lonely, very sad. She said, 'I know, it's often like that at the beginning. But it gets better.' Generally I am sceptical when people say this – that *it gets better* – but I liked this woman: I trusted her. Her daughter was pregnant with twins. As soon as the woman told me this, I warmed to her deeply. Before she left, she asked about my birth experience – for her daughter, you see, she'd like to know. I told her what I could remember. Worried by my ordeal, she assured me that her daughter had already decided to have a planned caesarean. 'Good,' I said, 'that's good.'

'Unfortunately,' she said, 'our charity is underfunded and under-staffed.' That summer, the summer of 2018, they had fewer women working with them than they would like, so it might, she said, take a long while to find a mother who could visit me once a week and help support me with the twins, but she, the manager, would come visit for an hour every week until she found someone. Whenever this woman came to visit during the month of Ramadan I felt safe. I felt secure. I felt seen.

It was important, according to Grace, to contextualise my life. Little by little, over the first month of therapy, I narrated that I was born in Los Angeles thirty-two years ago, the eldest of eight children, when my mother was only twenty-three, and that in her fecundity, my mother was different to the other mothers, there was a wilderness about her. She did not play games or bake cookies after school or help with homework or spend hours teaching me to read. More often than not, she was nursing a baby with her nose in a book, or pregnant and writing novels; and when not nursing or reading or writing novels or gestating or giving birth, she was in a baseball cap and tank-top in the garden, planting bare-root roses ordered from a catalogue or breaking up rhizomes or positioning much-loved stones she had scavenged from neighbouring properties as borders for herbaceous beds. Throughout my life, my mother was sun-kissed and youthful and strong. Her beauty was striking, distinctly Mediterranean. Researching my second book, I found myself in the archaeological museum in Naples, staring at the *Portrait of the so-called Sappho* from the Roman frescoes in Pompeii. The likeness to my mother was so pure, so exact, that I was moved almost to tears. Those sorrowful, intelligent eyes! That slender, olive face framed by a halo of dark curls! This! This was my mother. I could not, I told Grace, complain of very much in childhood. My parents were good, and they were brave, and they were kind. I loved them with a ferocity that knew no bounds.

When I turned five, my family left Los Angeles and moved ninety miles north to a small town in Ventura County. My mother had recently given birth to a baby and when we first left the city for the countryside there was a drought. The earth was yellow, the trees shrivelled and brown. Undeterred by the absence of water, my parents bought a dilapidated house in a valley near the sea and set about restoring it. I rode my bicycle to the ice-cream store in town and played little-league softball and attended a rural public elementary school surrounded by orange groves and went to the beach on Sundays and became, of a sudden, an American child. Steadily, we multiplied. Grace asked specific questions, then, seeking specific answers. Was there a history of post-natal depression in the family? Had my own mother found birth traumatic? I told her that when I was eight, the fifth of us swallowed meconium in birth, and spent a few weeks with oxygen assistance in an incubator. He suffered brain damage during his delivery, and went on to develop cerebral palsy, and, yes, it was true that my mother struggled with melancholy in the aftermath. Though she never named it as depression, we knew, as children, that she wept, and wept often. Only after the birth of my own babies would my mother speak openly to me of her struggle: 'I was trau-matised,' she said. 'To this day, I have an absolute terror of birth. Emotionally, it took me years to recover. I'm not sure, frankly, if I ever fully did.'

A reclusive and family-oriented teenager, I helped my mother as best I could. I did my homework at the kitchen table, reading a book or cleaning up dishes while holding a baby: I never went out, never drank, never had a boyfriend, never caused trouble. At fifteen, bouncing a baby on my knee, I wanted things, badly. I was doggedly ambitious in my desires: a classic All-American Over-achiever, I became a Rotary Scholar, Senior Class President. At seventeen, I was accepted into Stanford University, and won a Ronald Reagan Library Presidential Foundation scholarship. After graduating from high school, I took a gap year to learn Spanish at Spain's University of Salamanca, and study the history of Islam on the Iberian Peninsula, and while I was in Spain, my parents sold the house I grew up in, and began to build on a parcel of land in the wilderness above Santa Paula. There they erected the house that later burned, and over the years that they built that house, they rented a cottage in the foothills of the Los Padres National Forest, looking out over the Ojai valley below. I liked it here: our neighbours were psychics and gurus, and whenever I came home for the holidays from university, I shared a room with my three sisters. I had the bottom bunk beneath the nine-year-old. My teenage sister had a single bed against a wall – *her* wall – decorated with posters, and the littlest of us slept in her own toddler bed in the corner. Two of my brothers shared another room, and the third, seventeen and desperate for privacy, claimed a windowless closet as his lair. I enjoyed this, living like sardines. I found the proximity of my siblings calming. When I was twenty, we moved to the house my parents had built in the wilderness north of Santa Paula, and the next summer, shortly after I turned twenty-one, Isabella, the eighth of us, was born.

It was bell hooks who aptly observed that Betty Friedan's famous quote, 'the problem that has no name', was:

> *often quoted to describe the condition of women in this society, actually referred to the plight of a select group of college-educated, middle and upper class, married white women – housewives bored with leisure, with the home, with children, with buying products, who wanted more*

out of life. Friedan concludes her first chapter by stating: 'we can no longer ignore that voice within women that says: "I want something more than my husband and my children and my house."' That 'more' she defines as careers. She did not discuss who would be called in to take care of the children and maintain the home if more women like her were freed from their house labour and given equal access with white men to the professions. She did not speak of the needs of women without men, without children, without homes. She ignored the existence of all non-white women and poor white women.

I am a Betty Friedan woman, as characterised by hooks. In 2009, I graduated from Stanford in the top 5 per cent of my class, with Honours and Distinction in my major, and moved, again, to Spain, where I completed a Master's in Performance Studies at a joint programme between the Catalan Institute of Theatre and Barcelona's Autonomous University. As the financial crisis deepened in Spain, I relocated to London and got my first job as a production assistant in the film industry. I was twenty-four when I began to date my future husband and to write my first novel, a Gothic thriller, on my commute into the city for work. I was twenty-eight when I landed a six-figure, three-book deal with a British publisher, and twenty-nine when the *Observer* ranked it as one of the top debuts of 2015. While this book never published in the States, and never sold well enough to be notable in the UK, it launched globally in seven languages, ranging from Japanese to Hebrew. For a while, I travelled internationally for festivals. In theory these were all things to be celebrated: I was a financially solvent, full-time writer in my late twenties, but when I returned home to south-east London, as the publicity cycle dwindled, and I began to write my second book, I stood on the platform at the station in Honor Oak, waiting for the train to take me north to the British Library, and considered jumping. An idle thought at first but the impulse was strong, and consistent, and began recurring, and this scared me. Maybe, I thought, things would be easier if I simply did not exist. I had never felt that way before.

And then, suddenly, one day, I did.

The questions Grace asked, if she asked questions at all, following admissions like these, were often simple and deceptive. Questions like: *What was your marriage like, before the twins were born?* I told her I had not been married very long. Only a year, as a matter of fact, certainly not long enough to have many opinions on marriage. I was thirty when we married and thirty-one when the twins arrived: it all happened so quickly. The babies were born nine months to the day after our wedding and I still could not get my head around this. On our first anniversary, in an act reminiscent of Miss Havisham, I had confessed to my husband that I still had not taken my wedding dress to the dry cleaners to be laundered. A full year had passed and all the sweat and blood of that day remained as if preserved in aspic. Horrified, my husband bundled the dirty dress, its hem still laced with pine needles, into its protective cloth bag and shoved it into the bottom of the babies' buggy. 'Let's go,' he said, 'at once, to the dry cleaners, during the babies' nap. ' And we did. We took the dress to be cleaned on our anniversary. When we finished, we went to the jeweller to collect my engagement and wedding bands. These had been cut off my swollen finger, with a tiny threaded saw, during the pregnancy, such that each ring split in three. The jeweller had restored these bands, and I felt odd, putting them again on my hand. I felt I did not recognise myself in them, and Grace asked me why I had felt this, reunited with such familiar and important objects? I felt ashamed as I told her what I had not told my husband. I had not, I told Grace, taken the dress to be cleaned after the wedding because I could not bring myself to touch it or to look at it once I had fallen pregnant again, in case touching that dress wounded my children. Throughout my pregnancy with the twins I had fought hard against an impulse to throw my bridal gown away. This was odd, because before my wedding I had loved my dress. I had taken the matter of choosing it very seriously. I had seen it as an extension of my identity. A reflection of me.

It had taken me a very long time to decide what to wear. I am a private person, and in the year before our wedding, I had gone to try on dresses alone: a furtive, solitary act. I focused my attention, secretly, on the other future brides who existed in a parallel, buoyant world – flanked by mothers and happy friends. The larger the groups, the more champagne flowed between them, and in the beginning I was jealous of their festive intimacy, of the glasses of champagne, of the bride, appearing demurely from behind a screen, a new dress hanging from her shoulder, peeking out at her companions, and asking, again and again, *What do you think?* I was jealous of their shared joy, of the mothers sitting patiently, of the friends offering opinions.

As I tried on dresses, I perfected a technique of disappearing. I lurked silently among them, studying the embroidery, the lace, the beads – none of which I wanted. I did not like my own body, which I avoided looking at in the mirror, and I did not want other people seeing my body either. For months, nothing suited. I hated everything. As the year ran by, the wedding day began to fast approach and I grew worried. Perhaps I did not need a dress at all? I suggested to my husband that I would like to wear a tailored suit like him, but he balked, so I fixated on haute couture jumpsuits I could not afford and despaired.

It was in this state that I went to the house of a Basque dressmaker, on the recommendation of a Spanish friend. The dressmaker's atelier was in a personal apartment on a leafy residential street in North London. When I rang the door for my first appointment, convinced I had got the address wrong, the dressmaker came to the door smiling. She was heavily pregnant, about my age, and made me a cup of tea in her kitchen, which was filled with the spoils of a recent shopping trip – unboxed baby bottles, tiny diapers, pacifiers and bibs. The pregnant dressmaker led me to her living room, filled with gauzy, beautiful things, sat me in a chair, and asked me questions. I explained I was having a midsummer wedding, in Spain, on the island of Menorca, and that it was an informal evening affair, with the ceremony leading straight to dinner. She listened for a while and then sprung up from her chair, rummaging through her treasure, stopping occasionally, a hand to her back, apologising for catching her breath. The baby, she explained, was due in a number of days. Taking a seat, she encouraged me to browse. I felt tremendously shy. I moved about her converted living room, looking at the dresses hanging against the wall, and as I did she watched me, quietly, until, finally, she got up in excitement and pulled from the rack a simple slip in cream silk. This she suggested pairing with a matching removable silk jacket for the ceremony, entirely plain, boat-necked, three-quarter-length sleeves, pearl buttons clasping up the back. The jacket reminded me of something my great-grandmother might have worn in the thirties, but in its minimalism, it was also wonderfully modern. She held it up to me, pregnant and beautiful, and said, 'This was made for you.' Perhaps it was, perhaps not. But I liked her, and I liked her pregnant belly, and I was tired of dresses, so I agreed.

The next time I visited the dressmaker's home, she opened

the door holding her sleeping baby. I asked her about the birth and what the baby was called, and as the dressmaker spoke she kissed her daughter tenderly. It was deep winter, the floor was cold and the dressmaker apologised as she drew the cloth blinds shut around the makeshift fitting room with one hand, her baby snug on her chest. Behind the curtain, I shrugged off my clothes, and stood, shivering, in my underwear, facing an empty body in a narrow mirror. Suddenly I felt a great absence, naked and barefoot on the cold hardwood floor; a yearning that I did not understand. Slipping on my dress, I walked gingerly to the centre of the room, as the dressmaker called to someone else in her apartment who came up the stairs, another young Spanish woman who soon stood at the door smiling. The dressmaker passed her friend the baby, stuck pins in her mouth and came towards me. She pushed the fabric on my body into place, tightening the bodice, adjusting the hem, and as she did so, I did not look into the mirror as I was supposed to: I looked over the dressmaker's shoulder, at the baby who sat content-edly in the arms of the dressmaker's friend. The child was alert now, watching her mother work. As she held the baby, the dressmaker's friend shifted her weight rhythmically, bouncing slightly from side to side.

When I came again to see the dressmaker, four weeks before my wedding day, the dressmaker's daughter played on the floor with a rattle and I slipped the dress on, helped by the dressmaker, now flanked by a tailor, and, 'Oh.' The dressmaker tugged at the strap, ran her finger along the cloth draped over my breast, making a clicking sound of disap-proval with her tongue. The jacket fit tighter on my bust than she had expected. She asked the tailor if there was time to correct the measurements. The tailor said yes, but only once more – I found myself in a quandary: I had not told anyone except my husband for a month, but now, here, in the dressmaker's atelier, perhaps it was important. 'I'm pregnant,' I said to the dressmaker and her tailor, and the words were powerful, I felt myself transformed. Joy filled the room, the women laughed, they clapped their hands. 'Oh!' the dressmaker said and kissed me on the cheek and asked how pregnant I was and I told her, nervously, two months today. They spoke rapidly between themselves, enjoying the conundrum of my new body, conferring. What then to do? 'Take it out, here,' the dressmaker said to the seamstress, touching my bust, 'and *here*', a hand on my waist. As the dressmaker spoke, the tailor placed pins in the seams on the bodice, and together the two women adjusted the dress, so that it would remain loose at the waistline. I stood between them, watching the dressmaker's baby playing with her rattle on the floor. The night before going to the dressmaker's house, I had dreamed, vividly, of giving birth to not one but two babies, a boy and a girl. I had held them sleeping in my arms, and studied them, cherubim, tow-haired, pink-cheeked, and the clarity of this dream was so profound, so certain, that on waking I had turned to Callum and shaken him, breathless with excitement. 'Twins,' I said, 'I dreamed we were having twins.' I had seen two babies so clearly in this dream, and I had loved them so deeply that at eight weeks' gestation, in the dressmaker's shop, I felt an absolute, foolish certainty of their existence. Despite never having seen them on a scan, I imagined them learning to crawl, and racing through country fields. I imagined making their lunch boxes and taking them to school. I imagined them growing up and going to university and marrying. What would it be like as a child, to know that you had been present on your parents' wedding day in the womb? *There must be some magic to that*, I thought, *to the stories I will tell my future children*. And just

176

as I thought this, the dressmaker tugged on the shoulders of the bodice, and turned my body to face the mirror. 'What do you think?' she asked. The tailor fixed a veil to my head, and I remember thinking that the loosened, cream silk gown represented, in contrast to the traditional association with virginity, the secret promise of an unborn child.

After this session with Grace, I took the babies in their pram for a walk to the park near the health centre. On the way I stopped in at a bakery and bought myself a coffee and a sticky bun with hazelnuts on top. Pleased by this acquisition, I walked to the edge of an open grassy field, shaded by chestnut trees, and, parking my babies at an angle where they would not be irritated by the sun, left them to sleep in the shade while I tilted my head back and lingered on the clouds.

For a year, I had not thought about my wedding day at all. Not once since it transpired. I did not like being reminded of it. I had not made photo albums or hung pictures on the wall. My aversion had made me gauche. I had not sent thank-you cards, Callum had done those, and not consistently: he also didn't like to dwell on it. Friends had asked for photographs and I had promised to send them and then forgotten. I had not cleaned my dress or made mementos of my clothes, my silk shoes, my veil – *my veil*. This too would need laundering. I had bought it, impulsively, thinking I would have it refashioned into the baptismal robes of my unborn child. But now the idea of my boys' bodies touching the lace I had worn on my wedding day filled me with horror. I would not let my children near it; it was so tarnished by the violence of that particular event. As to the wedding day itself? I avoided mentioning it, avoided thinking about it, avoided even acknowledging that I was married. I had not changed my name, and never, ever referred to myself as a *wife*. I tidied everything away after we returned to London. Orders of service, place settings, photographs. Telling myself I would make a scrapbook, but I had not done it, would likely never do it.

And yet, I considered it a good wedding: it had been beautiful. In the park, seated by my sleeping twins, I saw myself, as I was on that night, one year before. A strange, ethereal, bleeding woman, drifting beneath the stone pines, moved by the private ferocity of her loss as her guests floated, nubile in the water, and I compared that old self at once unkindly to the woman I had become in motherhood: corpulent, milk-soaked, sweat-stained, numb. I felt nothing like that other woman on her wedding night. Yet I remembered things that she remembered.

I remembered, for instance, that four days before my wedding, on the island of Menorca, I had picked up my mother and my grandmother from their holiday home and driven us to a little salon in the suburbs of the seaside city of Mahon where a hairdresser had arranged my hair in the style I hoped to wear on my wedding day. The salon was sweet, and down to earth, and the woman who shaped my hair was funny and energetic, and I enjoyed introducing her to my mother, who had been for the most part benignly uninterested in preparations, but was now making up for lost time, obsessing over everything. My mother introduced herself to the florists and the hotelier and the caterers, and made last-minute changes to the arrangement of the venue, all of which were vast improvements. Preparations were progressing just as they should and my grandmother and my mother laughed as they sat across from me in the little salon, watching as the stylist did my hair. For eleven weeks I had kept my pregnancy a secret. But now that we had arrived on the island, I told everyone, everywhere I could, that I was pregnant. 'I'm pregnant,' I said to my mother, and my grandmother, and the ladies who ran the hotel where we were staying. 'I'm pregnant,' to the florist and the chef. 'I'm pregnant,' also to the woman doing my hair, 'my baby is due in January, six months after the wedding, can you believe it!' I confessed then to the hairdresser and my mother and my grandmother that I had made a plan to say 'I'm pregnant' to the collected guests in a speech on my wedding day. I watched my mother laughing with her own mother.

Chatter filled the small salon and from within a cloud of hairspray, and a host of pins, I thought: *How lucky I am, to be pregnant and marrying and spending time with my family.* I whispered to the baby inside me, 'You will not remember this, but one day I will tell you how we were here, together. That you were with me today, and that there were four generations gathered in a room, your mother, your grandmother, your great-grandmother, and perhaps when you are a little girl, or a little boy, you will be delighted by this story, that you were in your mummy's tummy on her wedding day.' And in my secret maternal love for the tiny life inside me, I felt tremendous hope.

An hour later, I drove my mother and grandmother across the island to the city of Ciutadella, where we visited another little salon, on another little back street, and met another local woman who would do my make-up on the wedding day. On principle, I do not wear make-up, ever, for many personal reasons, but on my wedding day I would make a singular exception. I confessed, with some embarrassment, to the women assembled there that I was a neophyte. '*Ay guapa*,' the make-up artist said, grumbling over my eyebrows. She demanded that she fix them. She could not, she said, work on a face as wild as mine. I watched her as she plucked at me. Her eyes came very near to mine. So near I could see each of her individual lashes. I studied her face, as she studied mine, and I listened, also, to my mother's suggestions. For an hour or so, I sat very still, telling myself not to be afraid of this stranger's proximity as the make-up artist concentrated in deep silence, adorning my face with the ritual trappings of desire. Creating a false front, a cunning, ceremonial disguise. When the make-up artist finished, she told me, in Spanish, to look once again in the mirror. I did not recognise the woman staring back at me, but I liked her. I liked her a great deal. I looked as I imagined a bride ought to look: arch, disdainful, vain. I resembled a matador, my hair swept back, my brows narrowed, my lips rouged. I was smooth and painted and untouchable. I felt like a work of art.

On my return to the holiday house, made up like a bride, I parked the car in the drive, and turned off the key in the rental car's ignition, and opened the car door. As I stepped out, I lost my footing as something foreign fell out of me: a strange peach-coloured ooze that ran between my legs, pooling thickly in my underwear.

That evening, as the sun widened, at the public hospital outside of Mahon the nurses handed me an empty plastic container and asked for a urine sample. The bathroom at the hospital had a large, long window, facing west, and I held the vial up to the light. The urine showed clear and golden but within it there were flecks of blood, swirling fragments of fleshy tissue. It was then that I knew. But I did not want others to know, so I wrapped the urine sample in tissue paper and washed my hands, and came out of the bathroom and sat next to Callum and told him not to worry. As I said this, I watched another pregnant woman exit the bathroom holding another little vial. She took her seat alone and in a gesture of subtle anguish akin to my own, hung her head over her rounded belly and waited for the doctor to call her name.

Partners were not allowed into the examining room during gynaecological emergencies. A nurse stopped Callum at the consulting-room door and said in broken English that he could not enter. 'Why?' he asked. Repeating the rules, she turned him away and led me to the consulting room, alone. There, she pointed to a pale blue smock, folded neatly, on a chair. The smock had a pattern of faint flowers. The woman asked me to take my clothes off from the waist down, to put on the smock, and to call for her when I was ready. I undressed, then, as I had undressed in the dressmaker's atelier. When I looked at the exposed pad in my underwear I saw that I had started to bleed properly. I called for the nurse, who came now, joined by a female sonographer. The sonographer asked me to lie on the examination bed, prostrate, my heals in metal stirrups, legs splayed. 'Wider,' she said in Spanish, pushing my knees apart. Then: 'Wider' again. 'Wider still.' I wriggled my bottom right down to the very edge of the table, offering myself up to them. One woman sat beside the bed, looking at a screen. The other applied jelly and something like a condom to a long grey wand with a bulbous end. The ultrasound, this woman said, would be internal. She warned me also, as this entered me, that it could be painful. Which it immediately was, her wand pushing higher and higher, turning round inside me. She examined every corner of my womb, hunting. 'There,' she said, to the other. I watched them watching the screen in silence. They listened for a while to the nothingness before speaking directly to me. 'How many weeks?' they asked in Spanish. 'Eleven,' I said. 'Then it died a few weeks ago,' one woman muttered privately to the other in Catalan, not realising I understood their secret language, and I began, uncontrollably, to weep. The woman holding the vaginal ultrasound asked the nurse to turn the screen so I could see. The sonographer holding the wand used the Spanish words for miscarriage, and I found it harsh.

'*Aborto espontáneo*,' she said, pushing the wand deeper into my body.

'The foetus has no heartbeat.'

As she said this, she pointed at the screen, and showed me a little silver shell floating in a sea of darkness.

The sonographer pulled her wand out of my body roughly, flicking a streak of blood on to the wall behind her.

'You can sit up now,' she said. 'The doctor will be with you shortly.'

The Menorcan doctor, who appeared soon, offered little comfort. I was, he said, to let things progress naturally. As he spoke I stared blankly at my blood on the wall. He was, he said, not a man who liked crying. It was good, in fact, that I was not crying, given that what I had lost was, after all, only a *malparto:* a bad birth. A malformed bundle of cells. Throughout, he made no mention of grief, or bereavement, or pain or haemorrhage or infection, gave no medical explanation of the normalness of my situation, made no remarks on the profound impact of loss, offered no statistics, or leaflets, did not, in fact, even prescribe painkillers. When I asked him why my husband had not been allowed to attend the scan with me in the room, he told me that women who receive information about miscarriages in the company of loved ones cry more, and their crying causes disruption to appointments. For this reason, the reason of medical efficiency, it was hospital policy that women must enter the consulting room during gynaecological emergencies alone. After this, he said nothing of any real interest, other than uttering a single empty platitude on the female condition. 'It will be,' he assured me, with great confidence, 'like a bad period.' This from a man who had never had one.

I, on the other hand, had had a miscarriage once before, when I was twenty-eight, and recently engaged to Callum, at a small literary festival in an English seaside town on the north coast of Devon. Again, I had been alone, and I had woken in the morning, in the hotel where I was staying, with a splitting headache. By the time I went into the green room, in advance of sitting on a small panel of debut novelists, I had begun to bleed. I bled through my talk. And I bled at a little table, signing copies of the novel I had written. I bled over lunch with an academic, and at the hotel when I collected my bags and on the rickety old train that chuntered across green hills, travelling with another debut novelist, who was working, she told me, on her next book, a novel involving the ghost of Dostoevsky. This woman looked down on genre writers, of which I numbered, and made it clear that she had not enjoyed sharing the stage with me and now did not enjoy sharing carriages on the journey home. After an hour we changed trains, and stood for a while on the platform making polite, stunted conversation, before she announced, as the train to London approached, that she wished to travel on separately. I was fine with that, and observed to myself, as we both pointedly entered separate carriages, that writers are not naturally convivial people. I sat on my own reading a book, and bled, quietly for the remainder of the five-hour journey. I bled a lot on that train, and over the nights and days that followed, and I continued to bleed, sometimes lightly, sometimes heavily, for two weeks. It was an early miscarriage, and the pain was not bad. The pregnancy was unplanned, and when it was over, I felt relieved and guilty for feeling relieved. Callum and I were only recently engaged, and at the time I did not wish to be a mother. I wished to write my next novel. What came out of me, I tidied away and flushed down the toilet, with perfunctory neatness, thinking: *What's done is done. What's dead is dead.*

This, though. This was different.

The night was hot. I could not sleep. Electric fans were positioned around the bed, and I soaked pad after pad with blood and the blood itself was darker than other blood I had seen before: it was black and thick and arterial and murderous. Just before dawn, in a kind of delirium, I said I wanted to go outside, to see the sunrise. Together, Callum and I went up on to the roof where I sat on an old plastic chair and held a warm compress to my belly, watching the sky turn pale. A stray cat without a tail rubbed himself against my knees. Swifts darted back and forth across the sky, sounding their dawn chorus, swallowing flies, and I remember thinking that I was not a mother but a mortuary, and I was a monster. Had always been a monster. I had a monstrous, murderous womb: my womb had suffocated my foetus. And then: the redemptive sky; the swifts, who never touched the ground, seemed to exist, solely, on air, shooting up and up into the sky until they disappeared; and that perhaps the baby who had been imagined, but would not come into existence, flew also upwards, and as I thought this I bled through my pad and through my nightdress and onto the plastic chair and when I stood up, Callum saw the pool of blood and said, 'This is too much, you must lie down, I'm taking you back to hospital.' He led me back to bed and went to call the doctor, but I did not want to lie down. The force of something else had begun and I got up and locked myself in the bathroom, and sat on the toilet bowl. My womb followed its own dark

189

logic and dealt brutally with the situation at hand. My body heaved. It opened and contracted. The blood was not simply blood: it was alchemical matter, the stuff of dreams. It contained, within its dark tissue, the clearly defined limbs of a tiny, embryonic creature, about which hung the invisible possibilities of a rapidly receding future.

I cleaned myself in the shower. Watched my blood swirl around the drain.

A bride, I remember thinking, exists solely for public consumption. She belongs to the collective and so too does the fate of her unborn child. *Next time,* people said, *you must rest more.* And while this wounded me, they were right: I had not rested. For months, I had practised Vinyasa Yoga. I had exercised frequently, done weightlifting. I had drunk, daily, a single cup of coffee. I had continued writing. I had lived a full and happy life and taken a warm bath every now and then, and walked for miles, and gone on a weekend camping trip with friends and eaten food cooked on an open fire and planned a wedding without a wedding planner and travelled by airplane to an island. Any and all of these activities, the collective felt, could have murdered my baby. Airplanes, another told me, were especially bad: altitude can cause miscarriage (not true). The stress of the wedding itself had been cast swiftly as villain. It did not help when I retorted that the rate of miscarriage has nothing to do with stress, and ranges from 20 to 25 per cent of recognised pregnancies (one in five to one in four) and that the vast majority – up to 80 per cent – occur within the first trimester, and that none of them have anything to do with the comportment of the mother, rather being an accident of nature, and that this is presumed to have been true across millennia of human existence. *Presumed* is the crucial word, as, of course, we have scant evidence. On hearing that I did not practise mindfulness, someone else suggested that meditating might have made a difference. 'Next time,' they said, 'you have to make contact with the spirit of the baby, you have to acknowledge it and invite it to stay here,' and they had touched their heart, 'otherwise their spirit leaves you.'

Pliny the Younger, writing of his own wife's miscarriage, observed with equal frustration:

> *The inexperience of her youth rendered her ignorant that she was breeding; so that she not only neglected the proper precautions, but managed herself in a way extremely unsuitable to a person in her circumstances. But she has severely atoned for her mistake, by the utmost hazard of her life.*

Of all unfortunate wives, Anne Boleyn, who fell in miscarriage:

The time had now come when Anne was to be again a mother, but she brought forth only a shapeless mass of flesh.

I greeted the guests who had arrived on the island and rented Vespas and wore large straw hats and sat in terraces on the marinas admiring the sea, eating sardines soaked in olive oil, as the nights approached the summer equinox. My midwife called, anxious, from London asking: 'Did you get my letter?' Lab work from the first hospital appointment had shown bacteria and protein in my urine. 'Don't worry,' I said. 'It's already dead.'

Shortly thereafter, two English friends of Callum, a poet and a scholar of Lawrence, beetled up the road on a moped, a bottle of red wine tucked in a wicker bag over a shoulder. 'Jessie!' they cried and showered me with kisses. I had never told them I was pregnant, but now I told them of my loss. I did not cry. Why should I cry? I was busy and important and had a lot of things to attend to: I went to Mahon, and looked at the flowers. I decided how fairy lights should be wrapped around the trunks of trees and where the dancing should take place during the wedding, and if refreshments should be served before the service. As more and more of the guests arrived, I felt increasingly responsible for their entertainment. I had asked a lot of them to come here, and they had crossed the world and had spent good money and I loved them. I wanted them to enjoy it. I wanted them to dance and be merry and I wanted to lose myself in music beside them. To be naked, and raw and ugly and wild. I wanted to disappear, to become invisible, to move unnoticed through crowds. When these things were not possible, I evaporated.

'So,' the vicar said, clicking his tongue, seated across from me at a little outdoor table shaded beneath pine trees, on the eve of our wedding day. The vicar, who I had not met before, spent an hour asking questions, running through the order of service for the religious ceremony. I am not religious, but Callum's family was, so I had agreed to a religious ceremony on their behalf – as a gesture of love – but now, after engaging with the vicar, I had begun to regret that choice. Before meeting us in person, the vicar had banned, with dictatorial control and very little explanation, the inclusion of a hymn I particularly liked by William Blake. Towards the end of our meeting, Callum excused himself to use the toilet, and the priest and I were alone. The sun shimmered behind him. There was a breeze, the air smelled clean. The vicar, who was old and white and missing several teeth, looked up at the trees and sighed: 'I'm not sure I really know what the point of marriage is any more. Do you?'

This startled me, but before I could properly answer, Callum appeared, head hung, walking back across the gravel. When he joined us at the table, he too said something unexpected. He told the vicar we'd lost a baby. Two days ago. That we were in mourning. He told the vicar that we'd kept the remains in a little jar but we did not know what to do with it next. Callum asked the vicar if there was any way, through the local church, or perhaps during the wedding service itself, that we could acknowledge the miscarriage of this pregnancy – was there anything, he asked again, that could be done to mark this loss? Maybe we could hold a kind of ceremony? A prayer or a reading? A poem? We had seen a *Guardian* article about a woman who had miscarried in hospital at twelve weeks and the hospital had cremated the foetus. But we weren't sure what to do with ours. 'Oh.' The vicar blinked. He had never, he said, managed such a request before. 'Let me have a think,' he murmured, 'and get back to you.'

I felt exposed. Two days earlier, on the morning of the miscarriage, Callum had called a doctor at a private clinic in Mahon who, hearing that it was my second miscarriage, offered to do a pathology test on the foetal tissue, and also follow up with a scan, and urged us to salvage the remains, and on hearing this, my mother had bravely fished the tiny opalescent being from the toilet bowl and placed it in a cleaned glass jar she had found in the kitchen, before concealing it, lovingly, with a scrap of linen, and hiding this, again, in a brown paper bag. This evidence we took to the clinic, a furtive act, full of trepidation, carrying my *malparto* like a scarlet letter or an albatross. Such is the power of taboo: once the being-which-was-not-a-being was in a jar, it was a thing, and in its thingness nobody, not least myself, knew what to do with it. When we arrived at the private clinic there had been a changeover in staff and the doctor Callum had consulted on the phone had long since vanished. The nurses at the desk refused to admit us, and expressing horror and disgust at the contents of the bag, sent us back instead to the public hospital, where I waited for several hours before attending a follow-up scan. At the public hospital the nurses scanned me vaginally and pronounced my uterus clean and reassured me that the discharge would soon slow. In desperation, I asked the nurses to please take away the jar, which I still clutched in my brown paper bag, to incinerate it, or dispose of it, as you would dispose of used needles, or blood-soaked bandages, or bodily growths or soiled paper on examining tables. The disgust on the nurses' faces humiliated me. They were horrified by its very existence, which they considered macabre, and said that on no account would they accept the remains, nor would they conduct a pathology test. When I asked why, they explained that they could not help with the disposal of the products of my conception as it had been expelled outside hospital, and that the causes of miscarriage are not investigated until you have suffered three, and so it was that I walked out of the hospital, numbly clutching my little jar in my little paper bag, and stepped into the blinding sun, feeling myself to be a criminal, the perpetrator of a tiny, private genocide.

'Why don't we bury it?' my mother suggested. 'Beneath a rose? Or an olive tree?' My mother liked plants.

But the rental we were staying in was not our house, and the island was not our home, and it felt wrong, leaving it here; everything about this felt wrong. Very likely it would have been therapeutic to have a ritual burial, immediately before the wedding day – probably we should have done it – but for whatever reason I could not face this. Somebody else offered to desiccate it in the sun, so that it would be easy to stow in our luggage, saying: 'You could take it home on the plane in a matchbox.' After speaking to the priest, I returned to this question of *what to do* with it and said to Callum violently that I didn't care what we did with the jar, but I wanted it gone, now, before our wedding, I did not want to see it any more. We could flush it down the toilet, or put it in the bin; all I asked was that I would never be forced to look at it again. I refused to handle the jar, to touch it; I could not bear to be in its physical company. Everyone else offered to dispose of it for me, but they too struggled with the *meaning* of the object, the lack of ceremony, the lack of guidance, and without being able to make sense of the object's *meaninglessness* after having been, for so long, so meaningful, they sought a kind of closure in its passing – a closure I did not want. So, as nobody was quite sure I was in my right mind, overwhelmed by grief, they sought counsel from the priest, and put the jar in the fridge for safe keeping, without telling me, in the hopes that the right solution – the right ritual – would present itself with time.

A few hours before the ceremony, the make-up artist whom I had visited in Ciutadella opened the box she'd brought with her in the bridal suite and turned towards me smiling. I felt the heaving. The sloughing out of me. I gasped, doubling over. I staggered to the bathroom, I collapsed over the toilet. Pain. Pain everywhere. Shooting across my abdomen. Ricocheting through my chest. I couldn't breathe. I saw everything. Blood. Blood. All the blood. Retching, then, certain I would be sick, and when I finished gasping and retching, I continued to sob violently in front of all of them. In front of the bridesmaids. In front of the make-up artist. In front of my sisters. I wept for what felt like hours: great, animal cries, and when I finished crying, I looked round and saw the terror on the clustered women's faces and apologised for having frightened them. 'I'm sorry,' I said through my tears, to my sisters, my bridesmaids, flower girls, the make-up artist. 'I am sorry.' The make-up artist spoke kindly to me, then she took my hands in hers in the bathroom and told me that in her experience brides often cried, a lot, actually, on their wedding day, and that it was normal to have nerves, and I looked at her directly and said in Spanish, 'I'm not crying because I am a bride. After I saw you, I had a miscarriage. I wore the face you gave me into hospital, and throughout the night as I lost my baby. I cannot go through today looking at the same face. Please, if you can change anything, change everything. I do not wish to look the same.'

In Ancient Greece, women walked the streets of Athens veiled and read portents of miscarriage in smooth wombs and deflating breasts and the emotional volatility of the mother. In Rome, it was popularly believed that a sudden fright, say, or sneezing after sex or smelling a strong odour or eating the wrong food could spell disaster for the unborn child floating in its mother's womb. Pliny the Elder, the Roman scholar (uncle to the Younger), lamented that the human foetus was dependent on the weakness of the mother: 'It is a subject for pity,' he noted, 'and even for a feeling of shame, when one reflects that the origin of the most vain of all animated beings is thus frail.'

'You are the first woman,' the vicar said, with some respect, checking his watch before the start of our ceremony, 'I have ever known to be on time for her own wedding.'

1815. Mary Wollstonecraft Godwin Shelley (herself un-mothered in birth) wrote in her journal, after the sudden death of her newborn daughter: *Dream that my little baby came to life again; that it had only been cold, and that we rubbed it before the fire, and it lived. Awake and find no baby. I think about the little thing all day.*

After dinner, on my wedding day, I made a speech. I'd intended to announce my pregnancy; instead, I spoke of losing a baby. Other women came and told me of their own experiences, held silent within, never mentioned. I was grateful for the strength gifted me by them. Their quiet meditations on bereavement.

I took solace in their fortitude.

Their *wordfulness*.

Their grace.

The dancing that followed the praying and the feasting and the speeching was explosive, a reckless frenzy. The night broadened, and as it darkened, the wine flowed and the dancing grew increasingly feral. Wedding crashers lounged at the bar: a woman in a skin-tight leopard-print dress and a man in pink shorts. 'Hello,' I said to them. 'Hello, hello.' They had slunk in from their neighbouring villa, following the music. I invited them to stay. When the dancing ended, and the bar closed for the night, people smoked cigarettes by the pool, dangling their legs in the water. It was at this point that one guest impulsively took off her dress and, finishing her cigarette, slipped out of her underwear, and into the pool, entirely naked. She swam out to the centre, a lone shadow. I found her carelessness intoxicating. The presence of a nude swimmer changed something imperceptible in the air. Time slowed. A dangerous energy hummed beneath the branches of the pines. As if in a spell, I took off my shoes and stood barefoot in the grass beneath stone pines and watched as one by one, in an act of collective revelry, the guests shrugged off their fine things and plunged naked into the pool. Callum, too, took off his suit and slid, diaphanous, into the water. 'Come in!' he shouted, and reaching up, touched my bare ankle. 'Come swim with me.'

'No,' I said. 'Still bleeding.' I busied myself, alone, gathering the dresses of bridesmaids left abandoned on the earth.

Ours was a blood rite.
A rite of passage.
From a sacred act of union to a bacchanal.

'For your friends,' the manager of the hotel said the next morning, lifting a sardonic brow as she handed over a bag of sodden undergarments, a pair of broken glasses, a book of verse. She did not pass judgement. I apologised, at once, but she brushed this aside. Nudity is not uncommon on beaches in the Balearics and anyways, she said, 'the English always do this. *Son pescados.*' Translated literally this meant that *they are fish*, but it referred, colloquially, to being heavy drinkers, *swimming in alcohol*. On the island of Menorca, the fact that the English were fish was universally accepted: to behave otherwise would have been out of character, and so it did not bother anyone, the hotel manager said, that our guests frolicked naked in the water. This was a relief, as I had woken in the morning mortified.

Goodbye, then, to my four sisters. Goodbye to my three brothers, and their two wives, goodbye to my grandmother and father. Goodbye to my mother, leaving us behind on the island, until: 'Wait,' my mother said, holding up her hands, 'I almost forgot.' And she dashed across the lawn, and into the house she had rented, and returned carrying a bag. She handed me this, saying, 'I did not know what to do, but you will know what to do.' She hugged me and kissed me and told me she loved me. Only when they were well and truly gone did I open the bag to find the bloody jar, wrapped in a square of linen, tied lovingly at the top with a black silk ribbon.

In the small town of Fornells, langoustine are fished routinely from the sea, and the fishermen's cottages are white and low to the ground, and the surrounding hills are harsh, blood red and barren. Callum suggested we eat an ice cream on the marina, and I followed darkly, resenting him, thinking of the bloody hills and the bloody jar with its thin black ribbon. I was so perplexed by the reappearance of this jar that I said to Callum that I was not sure I cared, really, whether we ate an ice cream or not, though I accepted his offer as a gesture of good faith. I was tired and I was sad, and not feeling very well, so I licked my ice cream solemnly and we sat together in the sun. We arrived sooner than we had expected and decided to wait on the marina before driving to a neighbouring village to pick up the keys to a cheap apartment I had booked for a three-night stay, before heading back to London. Dreading this flight, I finished my ice cream and said that I did not really see any point in returning to London for a scan that would no longer happen, and maybe we should just cancel everything and stay here and camp out on the beach. Before he could answer, Callum's phone rang and when he came off the phone, he said: 'That was the vicar. He's spoken to a crematorium in Ciutadella and gave them my number.'

'Oh,' I said, looking at the sea, feeling it was too late now for neatness. For discreet endings. For medical cremations of tiny beings sloughed out of bodies. No, neatness was impossible. Foetal tissue is not a thing at all, it is not a being, it has no legal rights, nor should it, for it is not a baby, it possesses no clear ceremonies, no rituals of goodbye to mark its brief existence. Death, I thought, is taboo in our society, and taboos generally exist for good reason, and miscarriage as taboos go is particularly difficult because the pain is borne solely by the woman, so private, deep, inarticulate and under-explored that it lacks clear avenues to healing. Besides, I had looked at the jar closely and the blood was now nothing more than blood, and had decayed beyond salvation, and needed to be planted, like a tree, or scattered among dry rocks like the miscarried kids of wild goats or be released into the waterways beneath the city, and be allowed like any other unrealised dream to disappear.

I said none of these things aloud to Callum, walking with him arm in arm around the marina, looking at the fishing boats. Saying, instead, 'How strange,' of the blood-red hills in the distance and the bone-white village and the flat, endless sea. When we arrived at our rented apartment in a modern condominium complex in those very hills, I knew with visceral intensity that I hated the colour of the earth in this place and the hills and their proximity, and the dark, grim bedroom with its unclean sheets. I was about to sink into a deep depression when Callum heard familiar English voices at the door, and leapt up.

'Is that ...?' he said, flinging our door wide, and it was!

'Hello! Hello! Hello!' our friends called out and when Callum shouted for me to come I saw three familiar faces, belonging to three dear friends who had travelled to our wedding independently, from separate walks in life, and connected over dinner and decided to come here, spontaneously, together, and by chance had rented the apartment directly beneath our own.

'Oh God,' they said when they saw us, protesting and blushing. 'We've got to go and leave you in peace.'

We laughed and said, 'No, it's divine intervention! Please stay.'

We hugged them and begged them not to leave as we weren't in a mood for a honeymoon anyway. We all agreed to go out together to dinner that evening and Callum invited them up to our terrace for a glass of wine, at which point his phone rang and he answered – sitting on the terrace in the afternoon sun.

'I'm sorry,' he said and we all turned and looked at him. 'I don't understand. *No. Ablo. Espag. Nol.*'

He handed me the phone. I remember the tone of that stranger's voice distinctly. The arch disdain. A guttural Castilian disdain marked by the distinct clip of an islander's dialect. The woman on the line spoke Spanish with the measured, imperious authority of a government bureaucrat and as she spoke, I could hear it, her lip trembling with indignation.

'An English priest,' the female voice said, 'called me this morning, and told me a very strange thing.

'He said he was calling on behalf of a young English couple, recently married, who are currently wandering the island with a dead baby in a bottle, hoping to have it cremated.

'Is this true?'

'Look,' I replied, in Spanish. 'I think there's been some misunderstanding—'

'*Señora*, do you or do you not have a dead baby in a bottle?'

'It's not a baby.'

'Well, then. What is it?'

'I had a miscarriage.'

211

She told me I had not.

'I have checked the registry of births and deaths,' she said. 'Only two women are recorded having late-term miscarriages on the island last week – foreigners, mind you. I cremated one baby, and my colleague in Mahon left the other intact – both babies returned with their mothers to their countries of origins to be buried. You are not one of these women, are you?'

'No,' I said, and she interrupted sharply.

'Then when did you miscarry?'

'Last Wednesday.'

'Did you go to hospital?'

'Yes, to Mahon.'

'That is not possible. No miscarriages were filed at that hospital last Wednesday.'

'Well,' I said, 'I had one.'

'*Señora*, how long has it been since your foetus was expelled?'

'I can't do this.' I turned to Callum.

I could hear her counting.

'Today is Monday,' the woman continued. 'If what you say is true, your baby's body has been decaying unattended for five days now. For obvious reasons we cannot now cremate your child ...'

'It is not a child,' I protested.

'... primarily because the hospital in Mahon has no record of your miscarriage, and so we cannot be certain you are telling the truth. Even if you are telling the truth the body has decayed now for far too long, and it is dangerous.'

I tried to explain precisely what had happened, but she again interrupted.

'None of this matters.'

Not the gestational age of the foetus (which meant the

jurisdiction she later referred to did not apply), nor the events that transpired before the wedding.

'At its core, it is the hospital's fault,' she said. 'And I will make a note of this, and reprimand them accordingly, but even though it was the hospital's fault, you must correct it. What you have done is illegal, in this country, my dear, and you must now go at once and hand over your dead baby to the police and you must declare yourself to the Judge at Alaior and he will decide how to handle your case.'

Nothing I could say would convince the imperious voice on the phone that I was not some foreign lunatic, destined for the tabloids, a murderous mother who had done the unthinkable to her unborn child.

'I am an officer of the law,' she finished, 'and if you dispose of any evidence before seeing the Judge at Alaior, you will have committed a punishable offence and you will be arrested and prosecuted for your crime.'

We did not go to the Judge at Alaior. Instead, Callum called the British Consul and spoke to a lawyer there who said that my goodness, the whole thing was terribly unorthodox and bizarre, adding that not once in his career had he encountered a situation like this but on *no* account should we go to the police or the Judge at Alaior, instead the British Consul would make an appointment for us at once with the Civil Registry in Mahon and the officials there would tell us what to do and how to respond.

Obeying instruction, we took our bloody jar back to the car, and drove to a severe edifice on the outskirts of Mahon, protected by armed police, where, at the appointed hour, we were ushered into the office of a female civil servant to whom we explained precisely what had happened at the hospital. As I spoke, I looked at the drawings behind the woman's desk – bright, happy drawings, clearly made by her young children.

Mama, one said, *I love you.*

I told this woman of the wedding, and of my family, and the woman at the crematorium, and the Judge at Alaior, and showed her my red NHS birth file which proved, without a shadow of doubt, that the foetus was only eleven weeks old when I miscarried, repeating: 'We absolutely do not have a dead baby in a bottle.' And at this point, looking at my file, she threw up her hands and said, 'This is a nothing,' and shook her head in an expression of disbelief.

'There is no need to record a death. You have done nothing wrong. All this,' she waved her hand, 'is a storm in a teacup. '

Someone had inadvertently given the wrong information to the woman from the crematorium. The woman from the crematorium had subsequently come to the conclusion that we had a dead baby beyond twenty-four weeks' gestation in our possession, which we had preserved, in a macabre and disturbing fashion. If this was the case, our crime would have been very grave indeed, but as it was not the case the civil servant said she was sorry for us, angry, even, on our behalf. I admired this woman. She was the only sane person I had talked to for days. She put the blame squarely on the hospital. They should have offered us a surgical procedure or disposed of the products directly when we came back to hospital. She agreed that the miscarriage had been handled badly. She used the Catalan word *'desastre'* frequently. *A disaster.*

Like the woman from the crematorium, she was most upset that there was no medical record of us having a miscarriage in the first place. She picked up her phone and spoke to someone at the hospital who would take the jar from us and get rid of it. 'Or,' she said, coming off the phone, 'if you prefer to handle it yourself . . . Do what everybody normally does: flush it down the toilet.' When she said this she made a gesture, raising up her hands and sending her eyes towards heaven that communicated she carried the weight of the world on her shoulders and we were but one of a host of endless troubles.

By mid-afternoon, the jar, and its contents, had gone.

In December 2019, a few short months before the outbreak of the pandemic, a new study on the psychological impacts of miscarriage in the UK, published in the *American Journal of Obstetrics and Gynecology*, presented evidence that early stage pregnancy loss and ectopic pregnancies could trigger symptoms of post-traumatic stress disorder.

The study, conducted by Imperial College in London, and KU Leuven in Belgium, surveyed over 650 women who had recently experienced early pregnancy loss (at twelve weeks or less) or an ectopic pregnancy. The findings were staggering: one month after pregnancy loss, nearly one in three women (29 per cent) met the official criteria for probable Post-Traumatic Stress Disorder. Nine months following miscarriage, nearly one in five bereaved mothers (18 per cent) continued to have symptoms of post-traumatic stress. Despite the high prevalence of PTSD symptoms after miscarriage, at the time of the study's publication in the UK there was little existing infrastructure in place to manage or assess the psychological impact of early pregnancy loss on bereaved parents. Underscoring a need for change within the NHS, the study's lead author, Professor Bourne, noted that 'those with significant post-traumatic stress symptoms require specific treatment if they are going to recover fully. This is not widely available,' he added, 'and we need to consider screening women following an early pregnancy loss so we can identify those who most need help.'

Several years prior, a smaller pilot study, led by Dr Jessica Farren (first author of the 2019 findings from Imperial), had already concluded that women might be at risk of developing PTSD following early pregnancy loss or ectopic pregnancy.

'At the moment,' Dr Farren had told Tommy's in 2016, concerned that women with PTSD were slipping through the diagnostic net, 'there is no routine follow-up appointment for women who have suffered an early pregnancy loss.' She continued, 'We have checks in place for postnatal depression, but we don't have anything in place for the trauma and depression following pregnancy loss. Yet the symptoms that may be triggered can have a profound effect on all aspects of a woman's everyday life, from her work to her relationships with friends and family.'

Menorca is an island of standing stones, Neolithic monuments called *talaiots*, T-shaped megaliths, formed of two massive boulders stacked perpendicularly, and *navetes*, large religious mounds, resembling the domed hulls of upended boats. I have always felt drawn to ruins: I feel myself reflected among them, and when the wedding was over and the jar had been emptied and thrown away, we drove out to see them.

Modern-day scholarship knows very little about the ancient people who inhabited the Balearics during the Neolithic period and built their monuments to unnamed deities. Rosemary grows wild among the stones, alongside blue narcissi. In the burial chambers, archaeologists have found effigies to female figures presumed to be Mother goddesses. They often have two heads, or bird wings, or chevron patterns. I went to the museum in Mahon to look at them, and once I had studied the female figurines, I went back to the ancient monuments, and put my hands against the stones. The *talaiots* were old, mysterious, full of indecipherable meaning, and I loved them.

We had decided not to leave the island. We did not want to go home yet, and had been offered a place to stay by a kind Spanish friend, so each day for a week, after visiting the Neolithic ruins, we drove to the coast, armed with maps and backpacks full of sandwiches and water, and we would park and walk two or three kilometres, through ravines and along gullies, descending cliffs to the sea, and then, and only then, when I was certain we were well and truly alone, did I take off my clothes and swim naked in the sea. Whenever I swam, I felt my heart lifting. We had lost something, to be sure, but we had gained something, too. A certain freedom: a new beginning. I would not fall pregnant again for a while. I would return and finish my novel. I would wait a year, maybe more. We would focus on our careers and reinvent ourselves entirely. Throughout, I bled, but the pain soon eased, and I did not mind as much.

In the spirit of new adventure, on the day of the summer equinox, Callum and I set off early to Ciutadella, to join the city's famous midsummer festival, *la Festa de Sant Joan*. We left our car in a lot outside the centre, and, drawn by the haunting sound of the music, soon found ourselves in a crowd forming around a portly little fellow playing a flute, as he rode a donkey. The tune was otherworldly, and very melancholy, like something from a fairy tale, and I have dreamed of it often since leaving the island. Callum and I joined hands and ran through the streets behind the donkey. We followed the piper to a central square, where the landed gentry of Menorca rode their black war-horses through crowds of a hundred thousand. It was a violent, dangerous performance, reminiscent of a bullfight. I was not surprised by the brutality. Bleeding still, I liked it, the ferocity of the dancing horses, the machismo, the red wine, the cracked bones, the blood. It was not safe, this spectator sport, not for the riders, nor the revellers, nor the horses, who trembled under the eye of the sun. People died often, drunk beneath the horses, or on the roads. In fact, people died every year, during the *Festa de Sant Joan*, but no one seemed to mind or be worried, so the festivities continued, year in, year out, in the name of tradition. To an outsider, the sequence of events at the *Festa* felt chaotic, and random, but they were not. They were governed by local folklore and history, each act laden with symbolic meaning.

Under the scorching midday sun, sweat bubbled on the black horses' pelts. They reared up on their hind legs and danced through the crowds, they frothed at the bit, and every so often, as their tremendous weight came crashing back down to earth, their hooves landed on the shoulder of some man reaching up to the rider and the music would stop and the medics would rush in. Once this happened close to us: I saw the hoof come down on a man's body and saw the blood and felt sick when the horse stepped aside, and the man didn't move.

'I can't,' I said to Callum, as the music stopped. Loading the wounded man on a stretcher, the paramedics spirited him away to an ambulance. For a moment, perhaps a minute or two, a fierce silence overtook the crowd, and then the drums and tambourines started again – and the revellers continued to dance beneath the horses, reaching up to touch the stallions' legs and haunches and hides, as a dare, reaching, all of them, up to the harsh-faced riders, to the bitter men of earth and steel.

'I want to leave,' I said to Callum.

The ecstasy, the violence, the inebriation, the hedonism, the hyper-masculinity, the courting of death. Once these things had fascinated me, but now they troubled me. Together we abandoned the festivities, pushing our way through the crowd. As we fled back to our car, the riders and their horses came suddenly upon us, and with them the clanging of drums and pots and pans and the crowd that swallowed us whole. After the horses, a blizzard of hazelnuts, thrown by the fistful into the air. People ripped open hundreds of bags of nuts left on the streets and hurled them into the sky, in an evocation of battle.

I wondered, as I moved through the deluge, shielding my

eyes with my hands, why I had so wanted to come and take part in this mad ritual. Once I had loved such displays. I had been intrigued by them. I had researched them, and thought deeply about their origins. I had worked, at twenty-two, with a theatre company in Spain, La Fura dels Baus, which rose to stratospheric success in the eighties building on the tradition of these popular festivals. I had structured my first novel around them. But now I was not so sure I loved them any more.

It took us over an hour to push our way back through the streets and escape. I drove us home. In the car, Callum closed his eyes and slept. Fragments of shattered hazelnuts clung to his hair. Halfway across the island we neared a megalith I had not seen before, and on a whim, I exited the highway, following a narrowing road to an olive grove and a field. I woke Callum then. 'I'm sorry,' I said. 'I need to see them.' He walked with me into the afternoon sun. Together we entered the remains of a Neolithic village through a narrow gate. I sat at the foot of a T-shaped *talaiot* still bleeding from my miscarriage, and cried. Returning from the *Festa de Sant Joan*, standing in the ruins of a Neolithic village whose belief system and identity would remain eternally obscure, I wondered about the rites of the ancient, unknown people who had erected these stones: their rituals were, in all likelihood, no less violent and chaotic than the modern midsummer festival I had just witnessed. I wondered, also, how many women had miscarried and married among these ruins. I looked up at the sun, poking over the edge of the stone boulder, and looked at the line of cement binding the rocks together, a job done badly, without regard for antiquity, in the seventies. It didn't matter what they meant. I knew nothing concrete about these monuments other than that I loved them: I found them painfully beautiful and felt restored by their presence. I too was a ruin. Looking up, I heard again the sound of the swirling swifts. Moved by the constant presence of the swifts among the ruins, I referred to our lost child, in my diary, as *el falciot negre*, the Catalan for *swift*, and in the years since, have continued to dream of it this way, a migratory bird.

During my boys' pregnancy, the swift came to my bedside often in the form of a grief-stricken nightmare: a cloud of narrow birds, breaking through the windows, racing through our London apartment, screaming out a dire warning. Now, I dream differently. Always the same pattern of events occurs. It is hot, shortly after midday. I am sitting on my knees holding a little spade. The sun strikes the middle of my back. I see the wind rustling the leaves of the mastic tree, and the wet patch of blood, sinking into the red earth, and I hear the call of the swifts above me. Taking a fistful of earth, I cover the blood, pressing it down into the roots of the wild mastic tree, and say, simply: 'Thank you.' And: 'Goodbye.'

SPRING

*A*fter therapy, I develop a habit of taking my babies in the
pram to the local deli to buy pasta and olive oil. 'Ciao,'
Paolo always says from behind the counter, leaning over
each time to admire the bambini. Paolo is from Sardinia. He
lives in London and works at the deli, but his wife, son and
mother are still all on the island. Over the early months of
motherhood, he had warmed to me because I knew a little
Catalan, and the part of Sardinia he was from was called
Alghero, in the north-west, where they spoke a dialect of
Sardinian derived from Catalan. Later, when the boys are
older, Paolo will refer to them, in Italian, as i piccoli principi,
the little princes, and if he is in a festive mood, even during
the pandemic, he will smile at my sons from behind his mask
and offer them a macaroon each in a little cellophane bag,
coming round the counter to greet them. Paolo and I will
chat awhile and commiserate behind our masks and for a
moment, during that first awful spell of isolation, I will feel
less unbearably lonely. The most important strategy in parenting toddler twins during the pandemic – and always – is
being present. Whenever I fail to do this, whenever I fail
to accept the constraints of my exact moment, a cloud
descends: I grow bored, anxious, distracted. It is crucial for

our mutual well-being that I enter into the immediacy of the children's little universe: whenever I manage this, this being present, my spirits lift. I become less a prisoner, constrained by the tyranny of Coronavirus, and more a voyager, exploring the unknown. My sons' joy when their little disinfected fingers crinkle open the cleaned cellophane bags is catching. Their curiosity, unbound. They discover things in ways that humble me. Each new experience, for them, resoundingly full, uncompromised. I love their fascination with newness.

CASE HISTORY

A diagnosis is comforting because it provides a framework – a community, a lineage – and, if luck is afoot, a treatment or cure.

Esmé Weijun Wang

Wheeling my little charges into therapy, telling Grace the story of my wedding, I'd park my buggy in the corner, nesting the babies near the door. If they were sleeping, which they mostly were, I would sit on a wooden chair with a blue knitted cushion beside the buggy, and talk, mutedly, in fear of disturbing them. If they were waking, I would rest each baby gingerly on a muslin cloth, which I laid out on the plastic play mat provided by the therapist. I brought toys in my bag and arranged them brightly round the twins: coloured rattles, a rubber teether in the shape of a giraffe, a crinkly black-and-white picture book with a mirror. In truth, the twins never had much interest in these objects, preferring to study other humans. Grace would say hello and they would arch their backs, suck their fingers and swivel around to see her: they liked Grace. Or at least, they rarely cried in therapy and I took this to mean that they liked her. As she spoke, they garbled merrily. Cheeping and purring, the babies warbled at one another, kicking a bit, banging at a rattle. Having surveyed the room, they practised tummy time, or rather, I placed them on their tummies and they pushed up on their elbows, heads bobbling, and grumbled to each other crossly. Eventually, their tolerance of my interventions ebbed and they rolled back on to their spines in a solemn, slow rotation. There, back-bound, happy, they scuttled sideways until their shoulders touched, and, 'Look,' I would say. 'Look. They are doing it again.' As one rolled neatly around the other, it began: the joyous entangling of legs and arms. Precision was not their forte. The babies cuffed each other as their bodies neared, swatting at an eye, an ear, a mouth, a nose. They scratched each other's faces, and nuzzled roughly. At which point, one would shout, in rage, and I would separate them. But they did not like to be separated. An invisible tether bound the twins to each other. Placed apart, they drifted towards one another, tugged by a magnetic force. Perhaps because of this, when I remember the beginning, I can only remember them collectively, multi-limbed, an octopus. But here, in the stillness gifted by the therapist's room, with its blank walls and mundane furniture, that vagueness lifted, and my children disentangled. I saw them, then, for who they were: two fierce little babies with the same face. They blinked their dark and daring eyes, unfurled their little fingers, and kicked. I saw them then. They saw me too.

That August it was hot. 'My little one,' I told Grace, 'he takes it worse.' The babies had colic and had it badly. Colic was the darkness. It was the creeping fear of death. It was memories of birth, of bleeding, of compression and expulsion, of incubators and cannulas. For three hours every day – from four o'clock in the afternoon until around seven in the evening – Baby B would scream and scream and scream. I took him to the doctors and they offered nothing. I took him to my breast, and this offered nothing. Eventually, I succumbed to stillness, lying on my bed, a baby in the crux of each arm, waiting for the screaming to stop. My smaller child seemed to experience living as a threat to existence. If anything remotely troubled him, whether emotional or physical, he howled in rage and despair; he shouted into the night, demanding to be held in my arms, demanding his mother, his father, to come – to come now, come at once – and relieve him of his suffering, and when there was nothing I could do he screamed louder, desperate for help. I gave him my arms, but could not stop whatever pain it was that he was living with and so his screaming escalated and the night lengthened, again and again and again, until my own head was pounding and my own nerves were completely shattered.

My husband worked hard that summer, and generally was not home till eight or nine in the evening, and when it got bad, I would call my mother-in-law in desperation. My mother-in-law, herself a twin who had lost a twin sibling, would race to my side, full of kindness and good cheer, often bringing a pasta bake for our supper. 'Little Darlings,' she would say, unperturbed by my sons' howling, and she'd pick the babies up and shower them with kisses, chatting in a bubbly way, about the Church – 'they prayed for you last Sunday' – about her summer plans, and the family BBQ and the holiday we would be taking together in Cornwall, around her birthday, and I grew to love her.

At home, battling the heat, I would lay the babies down, naked but for their nappies, beneath their baby gym, and set the fan churning, and I would think. I would think through nursing, as the babies sweated on me, until everything was sticky and cloying, and as they nursed I'd think about blood and watch them kicking on the pillows surrounding me. When they cried in the night, I soaked muslin cloths in cold water and pressed them to their foreheads, and fed them, like this, curled up on my belly. All the while doing my best to remember – to push through my amnesia. Little by little, I pieced together much of the birth experience that had come before. I would arrive again at my next session with Grace and tell her, in my signature detached cadence, that things for the most part were going well, but that the day before, when I had run myself a bath, and settled into the hot water, and closed my eyes, I felt, suddenly and viscerally, the pressures of a stranger's hand inside my body, and an awful tugging – someone was tearing at my insides, yanking down and down. I had the impression of blood – my own – rising to the surface of the bath, and I had not screamed, I had not called for help, because I knew it was not real, and yet I felt it so sharply – that when I saw the blood and shot up from the bath, I felt I was looking down at my body from above. Rather than dismissing these experiences or prescribing me medication, Grace suggested that perhaps this blood, this ripping, this gouging out, was the true root of my disconnection from my children. She encouraged me to make connections.

When she spoke, she applied specific vocabulary to the phenomena I experienced. She used technical terms like: *Intrusive memory, dissociation, hyper-vigilance* and *arousal*. And they had power, the simple act of naming helped. It was like letting oxygen into my lungs.

I liked having names for things.

With Grace's encouragement, I went that summer to see the gynaecologist again for a follow-up, as I had been feeling a great deal of pain and was afraid of having sex. The gynaecologist examined me gently and explained that there were still exposed nerve endings in my cervix – in the areas where I'd suffered a second-degree tear and a separate episiotomy. This was the source of the problem: the ragged bits of flesh in my vagina, bubbling up around the stitches, had healed badly. He cauterised the nerve endings, again, burning the tissue until it was smooth. It smelled strongly as he did this, and when he had finished, he told me to keep it clean and leave it alone for a while and see if it felt better.

Soon enough, it did. Empowered, I began to venture out with the buggy, not just to see Grace, but to buy milk. After buying milk, I went for a walk around the neighbourhood. It was such a small thing to have managed – getting down the stairs with the twins on my own – but it felt good.

Bolstered by this new freedom, I rediscovered the women I had met in a mothers' group before giving birth. I did not know these mothers, not really, and they certainly did not know me, but we were bound together by a shared month of conception, and my fate worried them. 'You must come out,' they said, recommending an exercise class they did collectively in the park, where you can do squats with your pram and restore your pelvic floor. All of them had shed their baby weight very quickly.

'I can't,' I would say. Politely.

These mothers with single babies were kind to me. They came round to visit once, and invited me to join a class called Baby Massage. Feeling brave, I joined them at this class, which the twins, I think, enjoyed. There were stairs leading to the room where the massage class took place, and the maelstrom of buggies at the entrance frightened me, I was too weak to carry both children at once, and did not like having to leave one baby alone in the buggy, getting the other up the stairs. In order to attend the class I had to email in advance and check no other sets of twins were attending, and then the teacher would take one of my babies for the duration of the class, in order to make sure he had the 'full experience'. This was the only mother-and-baby class I attended and I went five, maybe six, times in the first six months of my twins' existence. It was nice, and the teacher was kind and alternative.

After the class, a little group of mothers went for lunch together at the pub, and this was, perhaps, the most challenging part. I could not eat and hold two babies on my lap, and as the mothers always had their single babies to attend to, there was no helping hand for one of mine. They ordered pints in rounds and clinked glasses, and since I did not drink while nursing, I found it hard to relate to them. They dieted together, and exercised together, and drank together. They talked, often, of all the things I couldn't do: they put their babies in a sling and took the Tube to art galleries and museums. They breastfed freely, one baby, in public. If I tried to do that it was topless carnage. They had picnics and hosted small gatherings, noting sadly, 'I'm not sure there's room in our corridor for your buggy.' They went, sometimes twice a day, to baby classes and playgroups and sing-alongs. They were happy. They drank beer with lunch and wine at dinner and had their nails done and wore striped Breton tops and read beauty magazines in their free time. 'I don't understand these other women,' I said to Grace. 'The more I see of them, the more opaque they appear to me.' I was jealous. I wanted, desperately, the freedom they had, or seemed to have.

But even they were struggling. 'Oh,' one mother would say to another, 'the mistakes I was making, and I hadn't even realised', offering advice from the sleep-training book she had read which encouraged her to abandon her screaming infant over carefully timed intervals.

Then, the confessional, in person, at the park: 'It was harder on me than him. I cried often.'

Another added: 'The French do it so much better.'

A collective hysteria soon took hold as WhatsApp messages blinked on my phone: *It worked!*

Comparing success stories at the three-month mark, then euphoria: *He slept through the night!* Followed by despair whenever dreaded sleep recessions occurred, or the first milk teeth broke through, and the night sobbing started and the sleep training began again.

'It's hell,' they whispered over wine, worried little darling would hear. Should I be doing the same?

Crying it out, a technique much recommended by other mothers, including my own, felt impossible to me. My home was too small to leave one baby screaming, and my heart too sensitive. Besides, I tried to explain, inexplicably feeling defensive – it's different for me. If I neglect one, hoping to force him to cry himself back to sleep, the other rouses himself and roars in protest.

But perhaps I was wrong?

On the recommendation of the other mothers, desperate for rest, I tried sleep training the twins, leaving them to cry at intervals. One baby vomited, out of stress, and I wound up sitting on the floor holding him, promising I would never, ever, submit him to that kind of terror again.

Around this time, my husband and I set off on our first family holiday to Cornwall. We would have four nights on our own before his parents and his siblings joined us, renting a cottage nearby. On the first day my husband joined the slip road on to a major highway driving west out of London, a familiar road, one I had travelled many times before – but as our car hurtled toward the oncoming traffic, I believed: *Someone will hit us.* Of this I was absolutely certain. *It will not be my husband's fault. A stranger will hit us.* I saw the point of impact, the metal body of our car folding inwards, racing towards my knees, and watched as I died and my husband died, and my children died. Over and over again. The vision came in waves, like a warning.

'How did your fear manifest physically?' Grace asked in our session the following week. I had started to hyperventilate when my husband had first joined the motorway. Half an hour later, he pulled over at a gas station. I got out of the car. I paced. I sat in the car with the door open and nursed my babies, pleading with him: 'Cancel everything. Let's just go home, now. Please, please, I want to go home.'

'Had you been able to explain, clearly, why you felt these things?'

No. Words had evaded me.

My husband tried to soothe me, promising to leave the highway, to drive only on surface roads: it would take hours longer but it didn't matter. We'd go slowly. We could spend an extra night in a hotel, break the journey often. It'd be easy, he promised, we'd spend no more than a few hours a day in the car. We set off again, winding along back country lanes to Somerset. I was a bad travel companion throughout: my anxiety made my husband nervous, and as a result he drove badly. Or at least, I thought he drove badly and told him so, convinced he was being reckless, that he was not taking enough care. He did not understand the risk; he was deliberately putting our lives in danger. He found this hurtful, grew angry. Seeing this, I tried to hide my feelings from him, but the fear was too great; it burst out often and I shouted many ugly things.

Suddenly we crested a hill, and I had the sensation that we were flying. Beneath our wheels, the road gave way; Callum pushed hard on the brakes but the car hurtled, unstoppable, down the hill, skidding off the road . . .

I shouted for Callum to stop, to slow down, and he shouted back that I was unbearable, that I had gone insane, and I started to hyperventilate again. Callum pulled to the side of the road and I got out of the car and paced. What was the matter with me? Callum apologised and asked me what was wrong, but I found it impossible to translate my fear into anything other than rage.

Unable to understand my paranoia, my husband became resentful. At night, the babies, who disliked change as much as I, were not sleeping. The next morning, tired, ill at ease, Callum shouted when I shouted, and cried when I cried. The next day, we spent a night in North Devon. The third evening, we reached the seaside in Cornwall. It took us three consecutive days to cross the West Country along country lanes, and still I could not stomach it, and neither could my husband. He announced that we would not drive home. His parents were coming by train the following week. They would join us, and afterwards, they would drive the car back to London. We would return by train. I began at once to feel better. It was only then I realised how much I had made Callum suffer.

Outside the safety of my home, I found myself unable to sustain the performance of normality. I worried at the beach; I worried at the holiday house. I would not let the babies out of my sight, terrified by a host of unexpected monsters:

car seats, dogs, sand, seagulls. I made everyone a prisoner to my own fears, and the holiday was not a happy one. My problems were as exposed as my stretch-marked limbs and, in being exposed, opened me to ridicule.

I related all this to Grace, a week after returning, depressed and ashamed. She asked if the repeated vision I saw of myself and my children dying was a hallucination or something more akin to a memory. I said that it was both unreal and real. In my fear, I saw vividly the exact moment of impact, a violent collision, the memory of which was perfect. Hyper real. Immaculate. I did not just see this impact. I lived it. I lived it in my shoulder, in my spine, I felt the sudden whiplash, my body lurching sideways and slumping back. I could not get the vision out of my head.

'Did you have any somatic symptoms during your pregnancy?'

'What are somatic symptoms?' I asked.

'Headaches, pain, nausea,' Grace replied. 'Physical discomfort.'

I thought for a while. Well, I supposed. Yes. Seven weeks into my pregnancy with the twins, I had started vomiting. Again and again. I could not stop. Once I vomited over thirty times in one day. I went to see my doctor in Lewisham. 'Hyperemesis gravidarum,' she said, writing out a prescription for pills to control the nausea. I was sick enough that she offered to write a note, exempting me from five weeks of work, until the end of the first trimester, but I told her I was self-employed and could write through the vomiting. I was wrong. The drugs had an inebriating effect and I found it increasingly difficult to concentrate. But did that matter? The vomiting subsided at the six-month mark. I came off the anti-nausea medication, but was never able to finish the novel. By day, I bounced on, round with child. At the twenty-four-week ultrasound, *polyhydramnios* – a condition in which a baby produces too much amniotic fluid – was detected around Baby A in the womb. Shortly thereafter, my family's home burned down. At midnight, again in hospital, protein in my urine, an infection that required antibiotics. Oedema next, and rising heart pressure: my hands ballooned to the size of baseball mitts and Callum brought me to a local jeweller, where a woman cut my wedding and engagement rings cleanly from my finger with a tiny butterfly saw. Which was good, in its own way; when those rings left my fingers, I felt I had rid myself of the past.

But did any of this matter? Grace said that it did. At the end of this session, she asked gently if I had any history of previous trauma. 'No,' I replied tersely, bundling my babies in the buggy. I readied myself to leave.

As ever, I had lied. Neatly. Cleanly. Without a second thought. Because? Well, why not? Things were better that way. All this digging at the truth: it frightened me. Memories congealed in my mouth. I found it difficult to speak. What if Grace asked me that question again? What if she pressed me? What if she said, *What happened to you, before?* It wouldn't be safe then, for any of us. I wouldn't survive. Maybe, next time, when Grace's session came around, I could just *not* go? *Do it now.* I thought. *Quit. Call her up. Say it's over. Yes, that's it. Don't go.*

In the next session, avoiding eye contact, keeping my gaze focused on the floor, I confessed to Grace that I had once been involved in a car crash. I glossed this. Attempted to move on. She pushed me deeper: what exactly had happened there? The summer after I graduated from university, the summer I turned twenty-three, I went to the Californian seaside with a friend. We were driving home from the beach, wearing only our swimsuits, heading down the main road of our town, when a truck ran a stop sign and smashed into the passenger side – my side – of the car. In a breath, the illusion of solidity evaporated, metal crunched up like paper, and we span across the road, slamming into the pavement. The airbags did not work, and the metal door of the car had rushed in towards me, stopping a hair's breadth from my knees, and when it was over I looked at the glass all around me, and wriggled my toes, which I could not see beneath the crunched metal of the door, and it was only then, looking at the glass, feeling the presence of my toes, that I heard my friend screaming. She was screaming, in her swimsuit, screaming into the broken windshield, screaming and crying and repeating: *Oh God, oh God, oh God.*

On the pavement, I saw the driver who had slammed into us and the firemen shouting and the poor driver too was crying and so was his mother, who appeared, out of nowhere, running down the road towards us, weeping – holding up her hands, screaming, 'He didn't mean to, he didn't mean to. My son is deaf, he stole my keys, he doesn't know how to drive.' And all the while the firemen examined my body, looking for cuts, for bruises, remarking on all this, remarking on my weeping friend, the smashed car, the poor, confused driver. I remember thinking that it was incredible, really, that I had not lost my legs that afternoon, coming back from the beach.

'Hello,' I said, to the fireman who helped me out, patted me down.

I should have lost my legs, but I did not. So I was fine. And I kept repeating that I was fine to everyone who asked me. 'I'm fine,' I said, to the fireman who called me *one tough cookie.*

But I was not a tough cookie: I was numb.

I insisted to Grace that this impact – this car crash – did not bother me in the slightest; that I considered it a non-event. I emerged unscathed, and put it out of my mind and, except occasionally, speaking to doctors, dealing with problems in my spine, I did not often remember I had been in a car crash at all, until now, after the birth of my children. Why was it resurfacing now? Before birth, I considered myself to be an adventurous person. Cars did not frighten me. But after birth I recalled the forgotten accident so vividly it was difficult to tell myself it was not happening, right now, in the room. It didn't make sense.

I'd never associated the crash with mortality. On the contrary, it gave way to personal renaissance, a fresh start. Impact brought clarity. I reinvented. Shortly after the crash, I took a leave of absence from my co-terminal Master's in Modern Thought and Philosophy at Stanford, believing I would one day return, though I never did. Simultaneously, by pure coincidence, a female professor from the Institute of Theatre in Barcelona with whom I had been discussing a grant application emailed me saying the university had a space available on its graduate programme, now, if I wanted it, starting next week. The tuition fees for the year would be subsidised, all I had to do was come to Barcelona to matriculate in ten days' time. A European dual citizen from birth, I did not need a visa: I had the flexibility to make this possible. The professor realised the graduate programme might not entirely suit me, the rush et cetera, the scrum of it all. And of course there was the issue of language. The Master's would be taught entirely in Catalan, a language she knew I did not speak, but the university would provide free language classes. And seeing that you already speak Spanish, Catalan should come quite easily, and we will allow you to submit your papers in English. In fact, for political reasons, the professor said, we would prefer reading English to reading Spanish at all. This was exactly what I needed: a clean break, an opportunity to get away. I packed a single suitcase and bought a one-way ticket to Spain with the money I had earned waitressing that summer. I knew no one in the city but I didn't care: here it was, an opportunity, finally, for a new beginning. I swore to myself, on that plane to Barcelona, that I would never, *ever*, be a victim again.

Grace grabbed at this word, *the word,* which I left hanging in the air.

'Jess?' she said. 'Why did you call yourself a victim?'

Several years before the birth of my children, at a literary festival in a European city on the banks of a broad and sluggish river, I was summoned to a panel of European novelists (among whom, at the time, I still counted). There, I was asked the following questions: *Your book deals in many ways with the paranormal. What is your psychological relationship to the occult? Do you believe in spirits? Do you not?* I was young and fatuous and attempted to use this as an opportunity to speak about the seductive power of the paranormal and the dangerous – frankly religious – effect psychic prediction can have on individuals, thinking of certain members of my family circle, who had recently fallen under the influence of a psychic and from whom I had become increasingly estranged. But as soon as I entered into this personal revelation, I saw the journalist's eyes light up and I stumbled. Time appeared to slow, the beating of my heart grew louder, the room skidded out of focus, and I was flooded, knocked off my feet, with discordant images and feelings. After an asphyxiating pause, desperate to direct the attention away from me, I said that when I was in the bath, I sometimes heard voices, which was true and also not true. I do not quite know why I said this – the statement fell nervously from me. As soon as I had said it, I could not unsay it. My response was simultaneously translated into French, Spanish, and Italian – and my heart was in my mouth. 'Really?' The journalist blinked. 'Could you explain?' I could not explain. The audience rolled their eyes, my fellow authors bayed collectively, sensing blood, and the panel interviewer, a lauded journalist from a notable paper, frowned in a way that conveyed, with immediate impact, that I had lost whatever battle I was fighting.

Ah, well, I thought. *You live and learn.* Next time, perhaps, I would do better. The day before, summoned to the festival, I had taken the train from London, and arrived at a faceless hotel overlooking a sluggish river running through the heart of the city. There, I had met my publisher and had been invited to an award ceremony for a novel of the year, and later, a celebratory soirée, a welcome party in a church-turned-bar in the city's historic centre. Alone at that party, lost in the throng, I felt crippled by shyness. Deciding to leave, I went outside to call my future husband when someone tapped me lightly on the shoulder offering me a drink. It was the Man of the Day: the prize-winning author, whom I had watched on stage during the award ceremony, a cat-like, muscular man in his middle years, who was, by his own estimation, very clever and very handsome, and in a festive mood, and he smiled at me benevolently, handing over a flute of champagne.

'You seem,' he said, 'to be struggling. These things are tough on first-timers,' he said. 'Come on, come back inside. Let me introduce you to the industry.' We shared the same publisher, and were staying in the same hotel, and as such he felt honour bound to look after me. He talked about his first novel, or his second, or his third, about his career before becoming an author, about the difficult years, when cash was tight, and audience was small. He asked about my work, my ideas, my themes, and I felt myself relax, grow easy. He seemed a nice man. I told him I had written a Gothic feminist novel, which was meant to be ironic – a pastiche of the genre – but had been taken seriously, for which I blamed myself. I told him I was interested in the motifs of the genre, but was not a natural genre writer. I told him I was struggling with my second book, that was meant to be the sequel to the first, that I had been working on it even this morning, on the train, that I could not get my central character to progress. I had a notebook full of ideas, containing my archaeology of thought, exquisite lines, beautiful gestures, alchemical objects. In isolation, each note was full of life. But placed together, the prose sagged, momentum petered out, the story died. What was I to do? 'Relax,' the prize-winning author said, 'enjoy yourself. Everything will sort itself with time.'

He and I were taken out to dinner with the hosts of the festival, where we dined with a straight-shooting American Sensation, who sold in the millions, the impresario of my publishing house, a large elegant man wrapped in a Hermès scarf who stooped slightly as he chain-smoked cigars and talked animatedly to my editor, an intelligent woman who tolerated my emptiness amicably. Amid their sparkling conversation, the prize-winning crime author continued to look after me, throwing questions my way. His attention felt pastoral and I took him into my confidence: I told him about my life in London, my childhood, my fiancé. He offered to help with my next novel. Perhaps we could resolve some of its problems together? When I arrived back in my hotel room, I called Callum, full of light. I described everything, the bar, the drinks, the dinner, the conversation on the way home. I had finally made a friend. Perhaps I had a mentor in this man.

The next day was full of lectures, talks and hawking copies of my translated novel with booksellers, and then another dinner, another party. After the disastrous panel I shrugged off my embarrassment and joined my editor, my publicist and the prize-winning crime writer at a brasserie in the historic quarter above the river.

We raised glasses to the crime writer's prize, and the recent sale of my novel to a respected paperback publisher. When the dessert plates were cleared, my editor, pleased with the camaraderie between us, excused herself from the table, explaining that she really ought to head back to the hotel early, at which point our publicist got up to go to the bathroom. I sat facing the prize-winning author. He leaned back into the leather cushioning of the banquette, swirling the wine in his glass provocatively.

'So,' he asked, 'when do we fuck?'

'We don't,' I said.

Mine was a polite decline, firm and sincere, resolute. 'No,' I said. 'No.' Also: 'Don't.' We had dined together, after all, and it was not a crime to be attracted to somebody else. But the negotiations continued. He was surprised, he said, by the intensity of his desire towards me, and it seemed a waste given the demands of his feelings, not to spend at least one night together. Preferably this night. Tonight. Our publicist reappeared from the bathroom, and ran through our schedule for the evening, which, it turned out, was very long. I kept a healthy distance from the author but his hands had a magic ability to find their way on to my body: opening a door, getting into a cab. The publicist whispered, 'I think he likes you.' This frightened me. There it was again: that flickering numbness. That lawlessness going off in my brain, the empty ambivalence. I asked him to stop, but he did not stop. After an hour, I began to feel sick. When we arrived at the party on the boat, the author grew more brazen. He took my left hand and turned my engagement ring around. Tugging on my finger, he said: 'What would it take to forget for one evening?'

These hands which were not my hands. These feet which were not my feet. This body which was not my body.

'No,' I had said. 'No, no, no.' But this word, to this man, at least, seemed prevarication, an invitation for more. Enough. He told me that in his culture, in his language, promises such as engagements did not mean anything. 'I know,' he said, pulling me close. 'I know you want it.' We had reached the party now, and I looked over his shoulder and saw, to my relief, the female journalist who had interviewed me that afternoon, the same woman who had said, 'What is your psychological relationship to the occult? Do you believe in spirits? Do you not?' She was standing with a group of young people at the bar. 'Do you mind?' I said, brushing the prize-winning author's hands away from the body that was not my body, and walking towards her, shaken. Wanting to scream, or sob, 'That man.' To explain my statement to her about voices in the bath, to apologise, to tell her how stupid and distressing everything I'd said had been. How I had been ambushed, by my own fear, by that man, standing over there, by that person who keeps touching me, touching my arm, my shoulder, my back, my rear. Stumbling in badly fitting heels, my hand went out to her, sisterhood and all that:

'Are you drunk?' she asked.

'No,' I said.

She wrinkled her nose. 'You look drunk.'

She turned back to her friends and continued talking. I went to the bathroom, put on the flats I had in my bag, wiped the lipstick off my mouth with a tissue. The prize-winning author stopped me on the gangplank. Catching my arm. My arm that was not my arm. 'You're leaving?'

'I'm sorry,' I said, 'if I gave you the wrong impression.'

He told me I'd regret it, that I was making a mistake, he had, after all, been so willing to help, but if I changed my mind – he gave me his hotel room number – I knew where his bed was. I walked back, alone, along the sluggish river, the currents of which were melancholy, dark, seductive. I stood for a while on the banks of the river, and fought the urge to leap – the urge that had first visited me a few months before, after publication, and now felt terrifyingly familiar, repetitive, incessant. Once inside the faceless hotel, I locked the door, took off my clothes and brushed my teeth. Then I did what I have always done after situations like these: I washed myself compulsively, under scalding water, scrubbing my skin, tugging the dirt from under my nails, ripping my fingers through my hair.

Each time I encounter danger, I am back. Back in the little shack by the disused abattoir and the rainforest. There are cattle grazing in the paddock below, and to the north, a living jungle. I live these fragments in the present, so I write of them in the present. Above my head, green birds flash red wings. It is the wet season. When he walks me through the forest, leeches cluster on my ankles. He takes me wading, deep into water. The snake, poisonous, swimming along the surface. There are so many leeches, when I emerge, covering my shins. I bend over and pick them off as they latch to my body. Some already leave thin red marks. I cry. He finds it funny. He says: 'I wanted to scare you.' The towns, beyond the forest, where we stay, are small and dusty. The local economy relies almost entirely on tourism and farming – both of which are in decline. The cinema is outdoors, and drive-in, the façades on the high streets are wooden, resembling ghost towns of the American West. The indigenous people here have been systematically assaulted. The land carries the weight of state-sanctioned genocide, the communities that survive forcefully moved to reservations by the sea. The governing population, like my friend and me, is white. At no point do I feel like anything other than the outsider, and yet my whiteness binds me to this settlers' place: I am one of them born. Racism is rampant and overt. I meet, in varying forms, the hero-adventurer: the ranch hand, the cowboy, the industrialist, the logger, the explorer, the naturalist, the idealist, the artist, all of whom stake their claim on a shrinking and legendary forest. The songs they sing and the stories they tell are the violent songs and violent stories of occupation.

In the jungle, I live in a small clearing, in a rudimentary guest house, half open to the elements, with a bathroom and corrugated-tin roof, beside an abandoned abattoir. In this place, I do not have a cell phone or a car. I do not have control of my boundaries, or private access to a computer. The nearest town is one hour's walk away, the nearest airport, a ninety-mile drive to the sea. Through my host, I discover laws of contrition and obedience. Of submission and control. When I make phone calls, they are rationed, and they are listened to, a click on the receiver: someone else's breath. When I ask to use the computer, they stand behind me, looking over my shoulder. They read what I am writing. If I write a letter to my parents saying that I am afraid, they write another, telling them that I am wrong, that everything is perfect here. And if you say that it is not perfect, well then: you are weak. You are stupid. You will learn. For we are making a better person of you.

For years after leaving this place, any time I entered into any sort of physical intimacy, a switch went off in my brain and I was gone. Men said: 'I cannot reach you.' They told me that I grew distant, silent, animal. That I *did* not want them / need them / feel them. That I exited the room. Those that did not care for me soon left me, saying: 'You are not fun. You are not free.' Those that liked me, worried. They asked questions I did not want to answer. Nobody hurt me again, and for that I was grateful, but if any movement frightened me, I'd break contact, turn away, cry. If I fell asleep in someone's arms, to be roused by a sudden movement, I'd wake in the middle of a scream, sitting bolt upright in bed, and this terrified people, my screaming. Each time I'd apologise. 'I do not,' I'd say, 'know why this is happening.'

At university, when I first openly engaged with my bisexuality and fell in love with women, unrequited, from afar, as soon as the attention of women fell on me, as soon as I felt the suggestion of physical contact, I froze. I was absolutely terrified of exposing my own body, and would tell myself that this love was impossible, not because I did not feel it, but because when and if a woman touched me, she would detect the numbness in me, and call it by its name, and I could not bear the thought of naming. Whenever a woman approached me lovingly, I'd apologise. I'd tell her that I hated sex. That as soon as it started I longed for it to be over. That I could not orgasm. That I was asexual, nonsexual: that I never masturbated and did not like people touching me. That I would never make anyone happy. I'd explain these things to the women I loved, indirectly, cunningly. I'd make sure they never confused my interest for affection, saying, in abstract, I will always be a better friend, a truer friend, than anybody's partner: that my body, down there, is numb. Completely numb. And here I tell a little lie, a harmless lie: 'I have always been this way,' I say, 'not because of anything that happened to me, no, no, no, but because the numbness in me is foundational. It is part of who I am.' It is the very essence of my character. I am a mind, not a body. As for pleasure? I do not enter those hidden places. I do not feel those hidden things. For most people, this is enough to dissuade them. I hurt myself, often, doing this, but the pain is short-lived. Once it is gone, I no longer care.

Callum is the one to break this pattern. When I am twenty-four, he reaches out and touches me. He stops. He lays his bare hand on bare skin, and notices the shift in my breathing. He listens. When I wake, anxiously, rigid, on the verge of screaming, when I absent myself, go limp in his arms, stare at the ceiling, rather than asking *why*, he says, quietly: 'Somebody hurt you. Somebody hurt you very badly.' He doesn't care that I am broken. He doesn't care that I am damaged. 'You are safe, here,' he says, 'you are safe.' Callum teaches me to *feel* again. He teaches me to *want* again. The love I discover, through him, with him, is redemptive, kinetic, pure. That does not mean there are not ghosts, but they dwindle, lose their power, grow increasingly obscure.

In the faceless hotel in the European city, where I had come to discuss my novel, I cleaned myself in the shower, and as I cleaned myself, I drew the anger in. I stayed in the shower until I was red and raw as a lobster and then stood, drying myself in the steam. Still, I did not feel empty, and emptiness was what I wanted. After that I continued to clean. I tidied my things and got my suitcase ready for travel the next day. I reread my schedule, texted Callum, who was asleep in London, writing simply that I loved him. Suitcase packed, the room immaculate, body washed, I lay in bed, unsettled. For ages, I stared into nothing. *No one is holding you hostage,* I told myself. *No one is coming after you. You can handle it, make it go away.* The prize-winning author had touched me in ways that were unwelcome but manageable. He was weak and he was petulant, more a nuisance than anything else. Besides: he had not hurt me. He was not the hurting type. When the prize-winning author spoke to me again, over breakfast the next morning, I was friendly towards him, welcoming, I asserted power over him, I cut him down in myriad vengeful ways. The only thing that mattered was sovereignty. To emerge unscathed.

Gathering my bags that afternoon, leaving the festival, and the booksellers and the faceless hotel, and the faceless city, a seed of doubt took root in my mind. There they were again, the old doors closing. Better to be nothing than to be exposed. Better to vanish through self-inflicted obsolescence than to be destroyed by some unknown menace – the immaculate predator, inescapable, omnipresent, lurking in the shadows of literary prizes. Anywhere I encountered sexual predation, a road evaporated before me. *Your fault,* a voice inside me said. On my return to London, I cloistered myself in Lewisham, hiding in a rented, one-bed flat with Callum, where I spent my days writing and restoring a desultory, north-facing garden with poor prospects and little charm. Two months after the literary festival, unable to write with any kind of clarity, I submitted an unpublishable mess of a partial manuscript and adopted a kitten on what would have been the due date of the baby I miscarried at my talk in North Devon. My deadline was extended for a year, but I despaired. I was a failure, a fraud.

From that point forward, I avoided authors and events and bookshops. That summer I turned thirty, and Callum and I set a date for our wedding. Frustrated with my inability to write, I announced to Callum that I had found a place to rent in Spain, near the village where my novel was set, and that I would go there for a few months with my sister, with the intention of getting a fresh start on a fresh manuscript.

In Spain, almost immediately, I was happy. My writing began once again to flow, new characters and new stories populated my mind, but I was not certain, any more, that novels suited me. On the anniversary of my first miscarriage, the idea of a baby began once again to swim in my mind. In my breaks from writing, I looked at wedding dresses online, and dreamed about the future. Perhaps motherhood was the solution – the magic bullet. Perhaps motherhood would protect me? Make the memories go away? Reveal some undiscovered strength, lying dormant within? *Yes,* I decided, standing on the balcony of the apartment I had rented in Spain, looking at the sea. *A baby. That's what I want.* Once I was a mother, everything, I decided, would be better. I would take back control of my body. I would be powerful. I would be free. But I was not freed.

Five weeks pregnant with my future twins, I went to see my GP in south-east London. She asked about my wedding, and told me she was deeply sorry about the baby I had lost – a pregnancy she had also managed. She took my hand, pressing it between hers, and said, 'It must feel very difficult now, but I promise it will get better.'

Anxious that I had fallen pregnant one month after a miscarriage, she sent me for a same-day scan at an early foetal medicine unit, where my husband and I were told that I was not pregnant with one baby, but two. But, the sonographer warned us, early scans often caused more anxiety than they resolved, and she couldn't quite tell what exactly was going on inside me, this early in gestation. She wrote on our notes, *DCDA twins*. In another room, immediately after the scan, a midwife warned us that one of our foetal poles was not likely to survive the first trimester, being substantially smaller than the other. We were to come back for another scan in two weeks' time, when the embryos would be seven weeks old, and we would know a little more of what the future held. In the meantime, the midwife suggested, it might be sensible to get some counselling in place. She handed me a piece of paper with an advertisement for a charity that offered bereavement support to mothers struggling with pregnancy loss. I had never been in counselling before, but decided to make a referral. Several months elapsed before I was offered an initial consultation by the charity and both babies had now survived beyond the point at which the others had previously perished.

Heavy with children, I took the bus to a small, dank building in an industrial estate in London's old East End. During the initial assessment, a woman who would go on to become my pregnancy grief counsellor asked me to fill out several forms, full of questions. One of these questions asked: *Have you ever been involved in an incident of domestic abuse or sexual assault?*

No, I wrote in the space provided, and handed it back to her.

The conflict between the will to deny horrible events, Judith Herman, the pre-eminent Harvard psychologist writes, *and the will to proclaim them aloud is the central dialectic of psychological trauma.*

When I first returned home from hospital after the birth of my children, a health visitor came to my home to examine my episiotomy. That this stranger was a woman brought some reassurance, but I was alone and my husband had gone back to work and my children were sleeping, and I was not sure what would happen to me. Together we went down into my bedroom. I stripped out of my clothes and lay back on my bed, with my legs up, and felt myself exit my body as I had learned to in the jungle as she clinically examined me, pulling back the folds of my vulva to look at the healing wound – the stitches, the scar. The cut was still fresh, still raw. 'But clean,' she said, pleased, looking up, 'and healing well.' I heard her turn the sink on, and run water over her fingers as she washed them. As I heard the water run, and the woman wash her hands, I saw the spider in the mirror again, and felt the running water over my own hands. Just like that. The health visitor turned off the tap. Dried her hands. I thanked her, blinking back the tears, pulling on my underwear and trousers. Together we walked up to the living room. I said goodbye. She left the apartment. I cried, then. I cried and cried.

Birth shattered me. Things surfaced which should not surface.

Ten days later, lying alone in the mint-green room, the anti-biotics dripping into my arm, my breasts turned to rocks, engorged with unspent milk, I dreamed I was back in the little shack by the disused abattoir and the rainforest. In this dream, which is not a dream, I could not move. I was trapped beneath a body in bed. A young man has forced me down, and forced his way on top of me. This person is naked and straddling my abdomen and his hands are around my neck, pushing me down, his face contorted into a mask of anger. 'Shut up,' he is saying. 'Shut up, shut up.' In hospital, surreally, awfully, I lived this: the overlapping of past and present, the hands clasped around my throat, the voice telling me to stop – to stop crying, to stop it, stop it now – because he can't bear the sounds, the noises I am making. Inhabiting this place, I gasped for air. I felt my body go limp, my mind float away. I lost all sensation in my skin, barring a terrible heaviness, the oppressive weight of his body. I am gone. When he enters me, I offer no resistance. When he finishes, he offers no apology. He does not name it. We do not name it. Asleep in the crumpled sheets, he returned, disturbingly, to a state of grace. Once I am certain I am safe, I retreat to the bathroom and lock the door. Even though the windows and doors are closed, the sound of nocturnal life outside the little shack is deafening. I wash everything, carefully, methodically. I wash my face, my hands, between my legs. I look at my reflection in the mirror, and see the reflection of the spider on the wall behind me. The red marks, crouched and menacing, a purpling shadow on my neck. It is in the unbidden juxtaposition of the spider's grotesque body with my abused skin, like some medieval omen, that I feel it: the shattering of self, the line being drawn up from my pubis along my meridian. No one else will see it, but I will carry this divide forward, always, my own invisible *linea nigra*, marking out the territory of the Splitting Place. The Then-Now. The Before-After.

When a midwife woke me after midnight in the mint-green room, as my womb battled its own affliction, she said quietly, 'You have made your hand into a fist.' And she opened that fist, and laid my fingers flat on the bed. 'You have gripped that fist so tightly,' she said, 'that the plastic end of the cannula has bent in your vein, and the medicine cannot pass through.' Now, once more, she'd have to change it. 'It will hurt,' she said, 'only for a second.' Tap, tap, tap. Out it came again, in another went. Another yellowed bruising, another puckered mark. Staring at the empty cot in the mint-green room, my breasts burst, and soaked through my gown as I continued bleeding, out through my underwear on to the sheet, too weak to change my pad. The blood was pinkish, greenish, brown, and it was ugly. *I am swimming*, I remember thinking. *I am swimming out to sea, in a sea of milk and blood*. 'It was then,' I said to Grace, 'that the numbness truly descended.'

A sharpness here, in the therapist's consulting room. Airlessness, gasping. Or worse, suddenly fighting for breath. When I spoke of these things aloud to Grace, I apologised. I felt embarrassed. 'Perhaps,' I said, 'I am making a mountain out of a molehill?' I told her I wanted these memories to stop, to go away, and not come back at all. It would be better, I said, if they vanished, or I vanished with them, rather than this constant re-encountering of pain. After all, over a decade had passed. I had come here to talk about birth and my children and yet, here I was talking about this – about this thing that had nothing, absolutely nothing, to do with anything.

'Why?' I asked Grace. 'What is wrong with me?' When I left that place, I never opened the letters, never answered the phone calls. I never wanted to see him again. As I recounted this series of events to Grace, recalled piecemeal, like dangerous shrapnel, I watched her frown. Had she frowned because I was over-dramatising something that painted me badly, that exposed me as weak? I thought myself weak. When it came to dealing with these matters in my own life, I preferred to avoid the subject entirely, because it rendered me incapable of free will, and I would rather not deal in the degradation. I refused, in fact, to admit that it happened at all. I would say to myself: *It did not happen. I did not go there. I do not know him.* In the aftermath, the terms one might use – *domestic violence, sexual assault, coercive control, unwanted contact* – all of that clinical and legal jargon, repulsed me. What had happened to me was so *unremarkable*, so omnipresent in the narrative of all women, why centre my life around it? Even now, offering the specific details, say, of specific physical acts rendered them sensational and I could not bear this – the objectification of my body – so I opted instead for euphemism.

And anyway: if he was here, here in this room, beside me, he would offer up an alternative version of events, equally compelling. Adding to confusion upon confusion, he would say things like, 'She told me she had loved me, even years after the fact', and this would be true. He would say I had my own agency, in the matter. That I had made my own choices. That he had loved me, deeply, and that I had gone willingly, with him, into the jungle. That he had not meant to hurt me. Perhaps, even, that I exaggerated the experience of strangling, that it was a playful misunderstanding, a line crossed, in haste, perhaps, perhaps, perhaps. All from another vantage point, true, true, true. But if I examined the past through the lens of my current perspective, I found transgression after transgression. For years, I have wondered if these memories move my former partner, causing metamorphoses in him also, I have wondered if he too had nightmares, tortured by his conscience. I have reassured myself that he has never hurt anyone else again. But what if this is not true? What if he has not changed? Perhaps, if he has not changed, he did not know what he did? Even here, I am kind to him. Ought I to be kind any more?

From the place of friendship, in the beginning, I had trusted him. Setting the boundaries of my own body, I voiced my fears, gave my explanations, told him whenever he pushed further that I was not ready yet, and whenever this did not work, whenever he crossed a line, I feigned at once an illness. A sudden headache, an upset stomach, now, time,

time to go home. For a few days, I would avoid him, and then he would send a letter, make a phone call, apologise, he needed me, he wanted me, it wasn't such a big deal really, other girls liked it, eventually, so would I.

In the jungle, I accepted subjugation, at first blindly, and then with increasing horror, confusion and resentment, made more vulnerable each day by the abasements that followed. I told Grace that every day, for weeks and weeks, I would be led down a dirt road in the late afternoon, to an empty house, in the forest, where *things* happened – an *education*, he said, of my own body.

'I do not have boundaries,' I said to Grace. 'I am incapable of saying no.'

He had begun first to be cruel, verbally, and then to take me by my shoulders and shake me, lifting me up as he did so, almost as a joke. Towards the end of our sojourn in the jungle, he took me to a vast, unpopulated wilderness explaining only when we arrived, as the car that had taken us vanished over the horizon, that we would have to traverse the mountains to a point where a fisherman would pick us up and return us to safety – without professional guides, without Ordnance Survey maps, without mobile phone reception. It was a fantasy for him: my vulnerability, my reliance on him, the scrambling over boulders and stones, the scratches on my ankles and knees, the exhaustion, the setting up of camp, my fear and my frailty. He told me often, and frequently, that he loved me, and yet he was often very angry towards me, and made demands on my body that upset me, and when we argued, he picked me up and shook me so hard that my teeth rattled in my jaws. 'It is your fault,' he said afterwards. I had provoked him. When we returned to the little tin-roofed shack between the rainforest and the abattoir, I confronted him and said that I was unhappy and

I wanted to leave, now; that it was over, that I had been lied to, manipulated. I do not like to dwell on this argument – the events which I remembered after birth – because I find it difficult to recall why he strangled me with any precision other than the fact that I was strangled. Of the strangling, I said to Grace, I am absolutely certain. Of the sex, before, or after, I find it very difficult to remember. As for consent, in the moment, I do not genuinely know if I did or did not say *no*, but then again, once strangled I could not speak. Certainly I felt *no*. But it was my fault, surely, if I did not say it.

Grace pushed me to reconsider. 'I find your use of language worrying,' she said. 'I would class what you have described to me as rape. But you have not once used that word in relation to yourself. How does that make you feel? Has it really never occurred to you,' Grace persisted through my silence, 'that you might have been raped?'

Rape is a violent word. To cast it from my lips provoked anxiety. I might self-immolate. I might commit an act of bodily harm. Neither the language of the quotidian, I said to Grace, nor the language of the legal had sufficient terms to describe the specific pain, the transgression and the shame, of such intimate betrayal. Mine, after all, was not the earth-shattering violence of the unknown assailant. It was the heart-rending violence of the beloved. Here again, I find a dearth of language. A place where there are no words.

I think of *Alexithymia*, from the Greek. Pertaining to a lack. A lack of words for feelings.

It took nine, maybe ten, days, I said, to leave the jungle after my boyfriend strangled me, which was good, because by the time I got on the plane, the evidence of what had been done to me had almost entirely disappeared, but also not good, because I had to negotiate my own safety, which required multiple unwanted acts of submission. Once I was on the plane, I cried the whole journey home. I cried in the airports, through transit and in the airplanes, walking down the aisle, I cried to the flight attendants and at passport control. At home, my parents worried about my depression. They said that I had changed. A friend of mine from childhood invited me camping. We'd go with his family to the desert. As we approached the campsite, after a long drive, I began to feel overwhelmed by fear. I did not know this place. I did not trust these people. My heart began to race, and I felt suddenly nauseous. I asked for them to pull over, saying that I was sick, but it was too late. I vomited as I spoke, into my lap, all over my clothes, and the shock on their faces when they saw this, my coat drenched in my own vomit, filled me with shame.

Years later, circling round, I wrote in my notebook:

To speak of where he touched me is not the point. It was rather the way he touched me, pushed himself into me. Smearing his memories across my skin. His fingers were cold, unkind. They left marks that were deep and purple, darker and more terrifying than normal bruises, not filmy yellow, but inky darkness, pools of darkness staining my skin as he moved over me. When I looked at my body after, it was as if a dye had seeped into me and through me so that when I washed myself, again and again, scrubbed my body, I could not remove the darkness from my skin, the deep blood-red, blue-black stains, nor the feelings that entered me at those contact points and seeped into my heart and my chest, so that my lungs filled with toxic violation and I felt myself suffocating again. It was my fault. My fault that I could not get clean. It was my fault, my weakness that my body had been so easily, so permanently, stained by his.

'If what happened was coercive, and non-consensual,' Grace said, 'which indeed, from what you are saying, it was, why was it so difficult for you, in its aftermath, to land on a clear terminology?'

For a decade, if not longer, I had distanced myself from the truth using allegory. I had fixed my past firmly in the realm of the mythological, became an expert in self-denial. And yet the iconography of rape, intellectual, alchemical, continued to obsess me. Palimpsests also, wax tablets impressed with writing upon writing. They reminded me of layers, the layers of fractured identity written over my own body. The visceral, brutal violence of my first novel. Philomela, who lost her tongue. The nightingale who could not sing (metaphor, obviously). All those dumb ideas about tongue-less-ness that I kidded myself had nothing to do with my own dumb body, my own muteness. The second novel I could not finish. The feelings I could not feel. The love I could not express towards my children. I began, all of a sudden, to cry.

Looking at the clock behind her, Grace handed me a box of tissues. 'I'm so sorry,' she said. 'We've run out of time.'

For many of the nights that followed, my husband came back from set late, and I bathed the babies alone. Running warm water over my hand into a bucket, I filled the little tub and checked the temperature carefully. A digital thermometer first. Dipping my elbow in, *just so.*

The bath was shallow, and the water was clear. I cleaned my children one at a time, settling one baby into the tub, shoring him up with my arm, while his brother chirped beside me in a bouncer, gumming a cloth book between chubby fingers.

Bathing my sons, tending to them carefully, I dealt in forbidden possibilities: that when a woman gives birth, or when a woman looks at her newborn child, she may, unwittingly, remember violent things. Ugly things. Unspoken things. Things other people have done to her, whether in the present or long ago, which she now associates with the birth of her child, of her children. Things that threaten to unmoor her. That might distance her from her child and render her brutish or numb or reduce her to rage or despair, or prompt her to commit violent, destructive acts of her own. This was so clear in me, and yet I had never heard of such phenomena.

After bathing my sons, I placed them naked on a set of towels and patted them dry. I apologised to my children, on those hot summer nights, after my confession, for the burden of my memories. I apologised for the numbness. For the distance between us. For the presentiments of death. For the fear I harboured in my heart. But the babies, who had no grasp of language, and lived only in the present, cared nothing for this. The colic had started and they were hungry. They were cross. They were wet. They were cold. They cried when I shifted their bodies to arrange their nappies. They cried when I guided their limbs through fresh cotton. They cried when I did their buttons, fast or slowly, it didn't matter, they always cried, and when they cried, I brought them to the little cots beside my bed, and strapped the enormous nursing pillow around my waist, and gently positioned them there to feed. Looking down, I could not see their little faces: my pendulous breasts obscured my babies from view. I examined instead, the stretch marks. Slowly turning from red to white. A thin network of scars, rippling across my chest like a forest.

SPRING

You have permission, I tell myself, in the week before lock-down starts, to grieve. You are allowed to feel things, to be overwhelmed. And you must try, in feeling these things, to remain in the discomfort, with your feet on the ground. It is okay to believe nothing will ever be the same again. These are not dangerous thoughts: they are rational responses to an emergency. It is okay, I repeat, every morning, putting on my sons' hats and gloves, fastening the buttons of their overcoats, worried now of becoming hysterical, by the great heaving sobs that soon escape me, it is okay to feel pain, to harbour terrible anxieties.

'Mummy,' the boys say as I march them to the park. 'Mummy sad.'

'Yes,' I tell them, 'I am sad.' I sniff and wipe my nose, hugging them close. I smell the tops of their heads.

'Sometimes,' I say, 'everybody feels sad.'

At the playground (the day before it closes), I play a game of peekaboo with my boys in the swings, and they laugh. They turn towards each other and gurgle a private communication between them. I can't help it. I take the glowing screen from my pocket, to check the news.

'Mummy! Out!' the twins shout, sensing my distraction.

They're bored of the swings and we go to play in the sand-pit. Together we build a mountain, or perhaps a cake, or perhaps a castle, and they grow enchanted by this endeavour, and I return to reading the news on my phone. Simultaneously one son pushes a hole in the sandcastle for people to walk through. 'Castle!' shriek the boys. And promptly stomp on the mound of sand, flattening it. 'Again! Again!' We make a sandcastle again, using only our hands. They put sticks in the top and stir. 'Scrambled eggs!' Baby A says. 'Breakfast!' Baby B says. 'All of these things,' I agree. 'And more.'

INNATE DISPOSITION

I am angry nearly every day of my life, Jo; but I have learned not to show it; and I still hope to learn not to feel it, though it may take me another forty years to do so.

Louisa May Alcott

The foetus in the womb; sketches and notes on reproduction c. 1511. Leonardo da Vinci.

An explanatory note, by the artist, scribbled in lower left corner, reads:

In this child the heart does not beat and it does not breathe because it rests continually in water, and if it breathed it would drown. And breathing is not necessary because it is vivified and nourished by the life and food of the mother ... And one and the same soul governs these two bodies, and desires, fears and pains are common to this creature as to all other animated parts. From this it arises that a thing desired by the mother is often found imprinted on those parts of the infant that have the same qualities in the mother at the time of her desire; and a sudden terror kills both mother and child. Therefore one concludes that the same soul governs and nourishes both bodies.

Hysterics, Josef Breuer and Sigmund Freud observed, *suffer for the most part from reminiscences*. I am no exception. Once opened, Pandora's box will not close. Past, present? They collide. I live somewhere between them.

Each week, that summer, I plucked memories up like pebbles from a beach, and arranged them neatly before Grace and my infants, marking thin little lines on the sand. How on my twenty-first birthday, my pregnant mother snuck away, complaining of a headache, heaving the huge arc of her belly up to bed, where she curled raw, in a foetal position, shutting the door on the world. How I went, secretly, to her room to comfort her, and stood in the dark, at the threshold of her room, paralysed by the sound of her weeping. Knowing in my bones, as I had known from childhood, that the anniversary of my own birth always brought this suffering on her. How when I visited my mother, two weeks later, and held my newborn sister and felt her tiny, wrinkled fingers grasp my own, I had said, 'She is beautiful', and watched my mother wince, ashen-faced, hooked to her IV; felt the pain radiating from her like an assault on my own body. How my mother had been twenty-one in 1984 when she graduated from Oxford and how I had been twenty-one in 2007, then a junior at Stanford, when I pilgrimaged back to that city of dreaming spires, after the birth of my youngest sister, determined to make amends.

'The only thing worth remembering about babies,' my mother had announced, shortly after the eighth of us was born, 'is that the advice changes every year, and nobody, ever, really knows what they are doing.'

As summer turned to autumn, and my sessions with Grace unspooled, I played with my children on the floor. I helped them sit up on their haunches, supported by pillows, and cooed at them. 'Isn't it remarkable,' I said, often, 'how big you've grown?' Their heads bobbled slightly when I said this, like little owls. Setting the fan in our living room to churn, I tickled their bare six-month-old toes. I sang songs. They grasped at my fingers, pawed at the air. *Bang, bang, bang*, one went with a rattle. I liked it best when they smiled at one another, when one baby flashed his bright, gummy smile at his brother, and their happiness caught in my chest, like wildfire.

'One more thing,' I said to Grace. 'There's one more thing.'

See:

Late, autumnal, English skies. Soft, stone-coloured.
Boundaries blurring at the edges.

See:

A narrow room. Not unlike the room I attend for therapy.

A single narrow window and single narrow desk and a single narrow bed. A small bedsit in a brutalist residential hall sharing a communal kitchen, with a plaster bust of a philosopher on the windowsill, and a computer on the desk in the corner. My tutor, a graduate student whose history I shall never know, and whose complexity I shall never understand, does not converse much, or pass niceties. For weeks, he has perched here, resting his bottom, lightly, on his desk, his back silhouetted against the single window, while I read my essays from a little chair propped beside his little bed. My head inches from his pillow. Reading my papers, I smell him. I smell him on the bedding, I smell him in the air. He has a bookish, monastic smell, and keeps his room fastidiously clean. I cannot fault him for tidiness. But his life, like the room, feels narrow, and between the narrowness of the man and the narrowness of the room, I detect an intense and oscillating anger. With the changing seasons, darkness has encroached on my weekly walk to this place, and it is the darkness, I tell myself, that makes me nervous. Not the click of the door, closing behind me, nor the position of my little seat near the little bed, nor the ritualised proximity of his body, nor his odour on the sheets, nor the direct, unflinching quality of his gaze as I read my papers out to him in the suffocating room.

'Sit down,' he says, gesturing at the chair, shutting the door behind me.

'Do you understand,' my tutor says, 'what I am about to do to you?'

Time is so strange in this place. It is stagnate and eternal. It is visceral and blunt. I confessed to Grace that I believed on some level that victimhood was innate in me, its roots lying deep within my nature, and while I had insulated myself from the consequences of my vulnerability – changing habits; changing my body; making myself, as I thought myself to be, ugly – I could not change this fundamental aspect of my character: that I was prone to abuse. That when my tutor said to me, 'Do you understand what I am about to do to you?', I sat frozen for two hours in that place while he raged aloud, seated in that little chair beside his single bed, my hands gripped around the stack of papers in my lap, body trembling, eyes glued to knees, and that perhaps because of this freezing, I have very little memory of what happened in the room and cannot put it back in order. When I try, I see only the plaster bust in the window, and the pooling of tears on the stack of papers resting on my knees, and the floral pattern on the dreary yellow throw of his bed.

Returning to this event, not unlike returning to birth, I recall very little. I know that there were moments when I was certain he would hit me. He stood above me, arms raised, hands stinging in the air, shouting, and it was at these points, when he was shouting loudly –'You think I am a monster' – that the enormity of his body swallowed up the room, and I believed that he would hurt me. One of the few things that I recall with any real clarity was the full weight of his power when he said: 'I can take anything I want from you.' That I believed him.

Lost for words, repeating these things to Grace, I looked at the faces of my children. I studied their minute lashes. Their tiny ears. Their sweet, pink cheeks. I listened to the sound of their breathing and found my own breathing. Even though, I reminded myself, again and again, babies do not understand words, they do not speak English, I worried that saying these words aloud hurt me, and in hurting me, somehow also hurt them. They cried suddenly, and I put them to my breast. I fed them, hoisted into place, and felt myself grow animal, opaque. I told Grace, as if it were a riposte, a reason not to care, 'It's okay because he didn't touch me.'

He didn't touch me.

He didn't touch me.

Relating these things to Grace, I stammered, I stuttered. I inexplicably hunched forward, squeezing my arms tight across my chest. Pressing my face towards my knees, I bowed my head and trembled, my voice sounding hollow and flat. I started. I stopped. I told her that I had known from the beginning that the situation was bad, that the environment was unsafe. I had gone, the first week, to the administrative office of the overseas programme and told an official there that I felt uncomfortable. 'The tutorial,' I said, 'is in his bedsit.' The official listened politely, before brushing my anxiety aside. It was not uncommon, they reassured me, for foreign students to find the rigour (read intimacy) of the one-to-one tutorial system overwhelming. Tutorials, they informed me, were often conducted in private homes. Going to a tutor's lodgings, and discussing papers in a personal setting, was considered routine. 'At Oxford,' they purred, 'we do things differently.'

The next time I took my narrow seat beside the narrow bed, my tutor presented me with an image that he had cut out of the newspaper: a small photograph of a white, blonde woman. He asked if I knew who the woman was. 'No,' I said, 'I don't.' He told me she was a British Conservative politician. He did not like Conservative politicians. He studied the little photograph in his palm. Apparently, I looked like her, the woman in the picture, which was unfortunate because he hated her. He asked me if I supported Bush. I said no, I was a Democrat. He placed the photograph from the newspaper on the top of his desk, next to his computer. I read out my paper then and we discussed it. The tutorial finished, and I walked back to my halls of residence, a knot of anxiety in my stomach.

Invitations followed. To lectures in London, or on campus. I declined. The sessions fluctuated in time, pushed later and later into the afternoon, towards evening. He was rigorous, challenging, enigmatic, demanding. He told me my writing could be better. *Make it better.* I had intended to study throughout the year at Oxford. Four weeks in, I withdrew from the overseas programme. In the seventh week, I asked to meet privately with one of Stanford's administrators. Each time I attend my tutorial, I told the administrator, I read my paper out in a little chair inches from my tutor's bed. I do not feel safe. I would like to have the rest of the term's sessions in a college at the university. 'Perhaps there is something you might do to help? I do not think,' I mumbled, 'I can face going back into that room.' I was told, ruefully, that it was up to the tutor's discretion to decide where and when he taught. 'He is a good teacher,' the administrator said, of my tutor, 'a good person. He has never, in my experience, behaved badly.' I was encouraged to stay the course.

'Only twice more,' the administrator reassured me, gently, looking at his calendar, 'and it's over.'

'Sit down,' my tutor said when I next saw him, handing me a stack of papers: every paper I had written over the term. A letter grade in each corner, marked in brown pen. Above these, my tutor had taken a red pen, and drawn a circle with a slash through it and written the letter F. First on one. Then another. And another. F. F. F. 'Do you understand,' my tutor said, 'what I am about to do to you?'

Circling round, I blamed myself. I told Grace how, the day before that tutorial, I had submitted by email two feminist essays on post-colonial literature titled: *Sexual Transgression as a Means towards Liberation* and *Extracting Truth* and *Expunging Empire: Torture and Ritualistic Cleansing.* Both papers performed close readings of scenes of sexual abuse. Because of the content of my papers, papers I would be forced to read aloud, papers that include close readings of erotic passages and ritualised molestation, I held myself accountable for what followed. I will learn that close readings can be dangerous. That citations can be dangerous. That critical theory can be dangerous. Because he will ask me if I *meant to*. He will speak about me as if I have seduced him. As if I have entered into a relationship with him. He will accuse me of igniting desires in him, and tell me that I need punishment, that I have deliberately disobeyed him. I will get up to leave and he will shout: 'Sit down.' I will sit down. He will shout that I have provoked him. He will come nearer, shouting, insinuating things. He will shout, very clearly, very distinctly, 'I can take anything I want from you.' He will point to the papers in my lap, and shout: 'Do you understand? Do you understand what you have done?' I will miscalculate the situation and reach for my bag, and say that I want to leave, and he will explode. He will tower over me, raging, screaming, 'I can take anything, I can take anything, I can take anything I want from you.' He will lose control. He will threaten to destroy me. I will cry. I will beg to leave. I will ask him not to hurt me.

'I'm sorry,' I will repeat. 'I'm sorry, I'm sorry, I'm sorry.'

Why do we suffer more in the abstraction of language?

'Future, past, future,' Franco Moretti writes in *Modern Epic*. 'A present pursued by the future, which drives it towards the past ... a "strange" present: unstable, over-determined.' Time, in this place, Moretti argues, the place of 'history in progress', becomes 'narratively interesting'. Was I *narratively interesting*? In this shattered place, the place of mothering? Was being *narratively interesting* any consolation? A woman who thinks elliptically, who moves forward in endless circles, who closes her eyes folding laundry and hears, *I can take anything I want from you*? Who knows, with unutterable shame, that when that man commanded, *Read*, she read.

The body in pain has everything to do with the language of the novel.

An erotic impulse, this tutor's wanting and not wanting. His shouting and not shouting. Through tears, beside his little bed. Words taken out of context.

I see her standing barelegged in her shift, one foot in the basin, waiting for me to wash her, her hand pressing down on my shoulder. I lather the stocky calf. She slips the shift up over her head. I lather her thighs; then I put the soap aside, embrace her hips, rub my face in her belly. I can smell the soap; feel the warmth of the water, the pressure of her hands. From the depths of my memory I reach out to touch myself.

'Please,' I say, crying. 'Can I go to the bathroom?' He lets me go to the bathroom. He stands behind the door. I look into the mirror. I see the tears. I see the face. It is not my face. I sob. He can hear me sobbing. When I come out, I ask if I can go home. 'No,' he says, 'Sit down.' I sit down. 'Read,' he says again. I read.

But with this woman it is as if there is no interior, only a surface across which I hunt back and forth seeking entry.

'Slower,' he says. I cross lines I do not understand, enter a fetish I do not sanction or comprehend. I am frozen. Obeying orders. The man across from me, listening. His eyes closing, face relaxing. To be denigrated for a thought.

'You,' he says, when I finish. 'You disgust me.' Standing up from my chair, putting on my jacket. Then: 'Wait.'

His hand on my arm. His breath on my cheek.

'What happened here,' he said, gripping my arm, barring my way, pressing his body towards mine. 'What happened in this room stays in this room. It is our secret. If you tell anyone, ever, what happened in this room, I will come after you. I will destroy your life. I will destroy your academic career. Do you understand?'

'Yes,' I said, 'I understand.'

He let me go. But I do not understand.

When my mother visited me in London, ten years later, she crept down to my room, and gently turned my sleeping babies in their cots, repositioning them on their fronts, so that their cheeks pressed into the mattress, and when I corrected her, when I said, 'Mom, you're not meant to do that any more,' she apologised, and said she had forgotten. That the advice on sleep had changed since I was an infant. Still, she worried. A baby, she warned me, will sometimes dream that it is falling. And babies do not like this, the sensation of falling. It makes them feel lonely, she said. It makes them feel sad.

The power of swearing oneself to silence is strong. Three days after the incident in the tutor's room, I was summoned to an office, at Stanford's overseas programme at Oxford, where a university administrator, *erhem-ed* and pulled their door shut with an ominous, shuffling awkwardness.

'Um. Er. Um,' they said. 'Something, er, rather unfortunate has happened.' A letter from my tutor had arrived. In all his years in the academy, my tutor had written, he had never taught any student so repugnantly mendacious as me. I was, my tutor warned, a compulsive liar: a manipulative and vindictive fabulist capable of wanton acts of destruction, a danger to my faculty, a hazard to my peers and my university. On this basis, the basis of my acute mendacity, my tutor had failed me for the quarter and urged my immediate expulsion from Stanford. He never wished to see or speak to me again. The administrator read out lines from the letter to me and scratched their head. 'Frankly,' they said, 'none of this makes any sense. I have worked with you myself this term, and his description of your character does not match my own observations of your nature. This view of you, it disturbs me. I do not, quite frankly, believe it. Trouble is . . .' The administrator sighed. 'I will have to take the accusations seriously. There will be an investigation.'

'An investigation?'

'You will have to tell us what happened.'

'What happened?'

'Between you two.'

A deluge of violent images gripped me, and my tongue turned to lead in my mouth, my body froze and I split.

'He told me that I had written over the word count,' I said.

'In his bedroom,' I said.

'He kept me there for hours,' I said.

'He wouldn't let me out,' I said.

As I spoke, I saw the face of the bust in the window and the screaming face of the man, and the tears, smudging ink on paper as I read, *From the depths of my memory I reach out to touch myself.* The real, petrifying terror that accompanied this splitting, the pain of which was unbearable. And after the pain came the numbness, and after the numbness came the absence of memory, and with the absence of memory, an absence of selfhood. In the splitting-place, my mind emptied. I floated up and away towards the ceiling. I felt hysterical.

'Nothing happened,' I said.

As I spoke these words, words I was not in control of, the atmosphere in the room shifted.

The administrator seemed uncomfortable.

'What do you mean,' they asked, 'nothing happened? He didn't ...?'

'No,' I said. 'He didn't touch me.'

The administrator asked me then to write my own account of what had happened in the room and send it in over email, along with the course description and copies of any relevant emails discussing essay length and all my essays for the term. Writing this account, much as I would after birth, I felt nothing. Numbness, in this case, proved quite useful. Because I was numb, I was empty. Because I was empty, I did not say the unspeakable things, and because I did not say the unspeakable things, I was believed. For the next week or so, my fate hung in the balance. I hid in my shared dormitory room. I refused to go outside unless absolutely necessary, in case my tutor found me, or hurt me, or stalked me, and I stayed there until there was a knock at my door, and a cluster of worried faces appeared, all peers of mine, a group of students. A belligerent man, they clamoured, came to the building, looking for you, screaming your name. 'We think,' they said, eyes wide, 'he was your tutor.' After that, my tutor was dismissed from the programme and my essays from the tutorial were sent for grading to an outside tribunal. I finished my exams for the term, packed up my things and left without saying goodbye. I returned to California, intent on reinventing. No one, I told myself (already adept at silence), as the plane touched down, need know anything about this. But, as one day bled into another, I began to shatter. Something *had* happened in that room. Something-almost-very violent.

Next time, I worried, *he will hurt someone.*

After confessing this to Grace, I found myself unexpectedly repeating the same story to my husband, over dinner when he came home, long after I'd put the babies to bed. I felt surprised by this sudden outburst. As I spoke, Callum looked uncomfortable. He too started and stopped and then started and stopped again, and shook his head. He sought something, something to hold on to, to make things better. 'At least,' he said, 'he didn't touch you.'

I recalled then the face of the first official I told on Stanford's campus, after leaving Oxford that winter, how this man also frowned, his brow knitting, 'Oh,' he'd said. 'Oh, okay, all right,' more for himself than for me, and then got up, and methodically closed the blinds on his office windows. I remembered the sound the blinds made closing, and my conviction, on hearing this sound, that what I was saying must be shut out or shut in. 'Okay, all right, okay,' the man had said. 'But did he touch you?'

So, too, the face of the woman at Stanford University's Sexual Harassment Policy Office, who took down notes as I spoke. 'No,' I said to her, 'he never touched me.' In my head, as someone who had been strangled, that fact – the fact of not touching me – made what had happened in that room somehow better, but the woman did not agree, and continued to use the word: *victim*.

'You are,' she said, 'a victim of many things. Of sexual harassment and threatened assault. Of abuse and coercive control.' His bedroom was what she termed a *hostile environment*. In his bedroom, she said, I had been scared, bullied, threatened, coerced and intimidated. I had been victimised. All of which, she told me, were serious offences, made worse by multiple failed attempts to report my tutor's behaviour to the administration. Because of this, the State of California required her to investigate what happened to me, regardless of whether or not I chose to press charges. 'And, by the way,' she said, 'I feel strongly that you should.' Her office would support me: she'd provide a contact for an attorney at the investigation stage. There would be a hearing. The decision over whether or not to press personal charges, she said, was mine. The terror roared up in me, and I said: No. I do not want a lawyer. No. I do not want a hearing. No. I do not want to press charges. No. I do not want to tell my parents. No. I do not want to ever speak or see or hear from that man. 'All I want,' I said to the woman, 'is for you to make sure this never, ever, happens to anyone else again.' The woman from Stanford's Sexual Harassment Policy Office shook her head and sighed. She said she regretted my decision but reassured me that she would continue to investigate my case, regardless of my involvement, as the assault I described was serious enough to warrant further examination, and the need for implementing safeguarding on overseas programmes was real. During this investigation I would have total anonymity. In the meantime, she recommended I seek out therapy. I made an appointment through the student mental health services on campus, but when it came to it, and I sat down on the chair, I remained entirely mute. I would not return to a therapist's room again until after the birth of my children.

The records kept by the university of this exchange are not substantial. They are delivered to me via Zoom, over the course of finishing this book, mediated by a pleasant young woman with a blurred background, who is thoughtful and kind, as she reminds me that digital copies are not permitted, nor am I allowed to record the session, nor am I allowed to have a third-party present in the room. She holds the pages up to the camera and says, *take your time*. My case report, a single page masterclass in brevity, is filled with acronyms and broken sentences. Fourteen years later, I am struck by the care, taken by the university, the tenderness in correspondence. The notes outline a minor investigation, ripe with the surreal idiosyncrasies of the recently traumatised, swiftly executed, with immediate effect. I am interested most by the silences.

For a few months, following the incident at Oxford, I had night terrors, panic attacks, trouble concentrating. I exercised less. Drank more. Gained ten, maybe fifteen pounds. My grades suffered and I began, in anger, to hurt myself. I made small, precise incisions on my fingers and thumbs with whatever was to hand – the end of a mechanical pencil, a ruler, a safety pin – deep enough to draw blood, and then, slowly, exactingly, I would squeeze out the blood and watch it jewel on my skin. I was very careful doing this. I kept the wounds on my fingers clean. Scrubbed them hard with soap when I finished. The narrative I wished to control was one of victimhood: a word I excised entirely from my vocabulary. Clean wounds, I reassured myself, healed faster than messy ones. If an experience bothers you, I told myself, cut it out. From your body. From your mind. Part of you may hurt while doing this. Hurting, after all, is only natural. If you begin to hurt, amputate that part of yourself which is hurting. Do it swiftly, with precision. Forgetting is better. Much better than remembering. If anyone challenges you, if they can recall the past, or worry, say, that you seem different or distant, cut them out also: keep going until there's nothing left. Finally, when the severance has healed, deny the existence of scars.

Sometime in late winter, or maybe early spring, two young women, both students at Stanford, approached me at a party. 'Hey,' they said, 'are you—?' And they named me, and they named my tutor. They told me they were part of an investigation. Our tutor had taught them last year, at the Programme in Oxford, in his bedroom, and he was, they said, volatile with them, and violent in his language towards them. They told me that my tutor had frightened them, with the placement of his body, with his eyes, that he was aggressive, unstable, vindictive. Both had reported him to the administration. Both had warned that he should not teach again. But their voices had not been heard. They wanted me to know that they had tried. That they too had said, *Next time, he will hurt someone.*

That summer, on a Stanford research seminar in India, investigating the legacy of non-violence and the crimes against humanity committed during communal violence in Gujarat in 2002, a student went to her room and cut off her lengthy hair. When she reappeared the next morning at the seminar, with her shaved skull, we stared as she sat down. Why, we asked, had she done this? She spoke at length of how the survivors' testimonies we had heard of the sexual violence committed against the Muslim women of Gujarat in 2002 had shocked her deeply, radically altering her world view. Rape, she said violently, happens everywhere, all around us. But it is not treated as a crime. If it is not treated as a crime, who is held accountable? Language must change. There must be consequences. Victims must receive an official apology and compensation from the state. Politicians and religious leaders must be tried. Punishment must be enacted. New policies must be put in place to protect women, and rape must be prosecuted at all costs. Gender-based violence, this young woman said, was a pressing social and political issue. Identifiable perpetrators of the mass rapes and murders in Gujarat must be tried in a court and sentenced by a jury. Without making these changes, without demonstrating to a victim that what happened to her *matters*, that rape is a crime, punishable by law, how else will she put her life back together? How else will she recover? *Nothing changes. Nothing stops.* This is why, the student said, she had shaved her head, cutting off her hair, the symbol of her femininity, in protest. We live in a world defined by rape. Nowhere is safe. And as evidence of this, in the seminar in India, the girl with the shaved skull began to tell the story of a scandal. Last spring, she said, she had been an overseas student at Oxford, where a female student, from Stanford, had been attacked by her tutor in his bedroom in the autumn. The girl, she said, had vanished, been entirely disappeared. She described the safeguarding that had been put in place after I left, of which I knew nothing. As she spoke, I began to feel sick: rumours had grown in my absence, and as they had grown, I had become a myth, a cautionary tale. The implication was now that I had been raped by my tutor. But this was not true, and as someone who had been raped, I wished to make this distinction. I wished to tell her I was alive and well and I am sitting here beside you and I am not destroyed. I am not disappeared. I am not a victim. I am *me*. I wanted to make sure that she understood this, that what had happened to me was nowhere near as bad as she said, and this is why I broke my silence, why I said, *That was me*, because I couldn't bear the implication that I had been raped at Oxford, after hearing the testimony of so many women who had been raped.

'That was me,' I said. 'That was me.'

The blankness then.
    The obliterating silence.

In the supermarket, I pulled the milk from the fridge, the butter from the rack, the bread from the shelf. I packed them neatly in the basket resting over my arm as the babies stirred in the pram, still sleeping. I sorted our shopping. Outside it was raining. Rain flooded down the peak of my hood, as I tugged at the ill-fitting rain guard, pulling steaming plastic over the hoods of the buggy, keeping the babies dry. Buses veered by, stacked with faces. I walked the avenue of trees, numb. I wanted to cry. But nothing emerged.

'I have tried, and I have tried,' I would later say to Grace, 'but I am incapable of expressing feeling.'

Sitting on the floor, shaking a rattle at the babies, Grace told me that my particular profile, my case history of sexual assault and sexual harassment, made me particularly susceptible to postnatal depression and post-traumatic stress disorder. She explained that the violence inflicted on my womb, in birth, echoed past violence inflicted on the same regions. That my body, recognising this echo, had set about to remind me: *this world is a dangerous place*. She said also that the violent recollection of rape in birth was not an unusual experience in survivors, that, on the contrary, the phenomenon of postnatal depression and post-traumatic stress disorder in women who had previously experienced trauma had been studied. That the acute numbness caused by the combination of birth trauma and the intrusion of other, associated memories into the fabric of my newfound motherhood was not unusual. It was clinically predictable.

After therapy, I retreated to the kitchen table, long after the sun had set, and my babies were asleep, and my husband had returned from work, and drank my lukewarm cup of tea and began my nightly ritual. I removed the plastic cups and bottles and suction devices from the steriliser and assembled them into a machine. Attaching them to the thin silicon tubes that dangled from the pump, I inserted my breasts into the suction cups and arranged the bra-like contraption with its large holes over my nipples, and began, as I always did, at the end of every empty, endless day, to pump. I recalled reading, then, something distant, something from long ago: that in 1795, in the old merchant town of Tønsberg, in Norway, Mary Wollstonecraft had spent three weeks in a little inn overlooking a bay and that she had travelled there with her nurse and infant daughter, fleeing tragedy and scandal. Before arriving in Scandinavia, Mary had attempted suicide, and in Tønsberg she spent her days tending to her baby and recovering, or wandering alone along the cliffs, or rowing out in a little boat into the little bay. Here, Mary too allowed her thoughts to drift, looking at the forest, or the glistening jellyfish in the depths of the currents, and she began, slowly, to assemble the notes for a book. 'It appears to me impossible,' Mary wrote, of drifting out to sea, 'that I should cease to exist, or that this active, restless spirit, equally alive to joy and sorrow, should be only organised to dust – ready to fly abroad the moment the spring snaps, or the spark goes out, which kept it together. Surely something resides in this heart that is not perishable – and life is more than a dream.'

I would tell Grace, the next time I saw her, that increasingly I believed that a woman's reproductive history could not be separated from the weight of the history that she carried. That mothers were not born. They were made. And they could be unmade. And that between the making and the unmaking every day was a struggle for self-definition.

SPRING

Flinging their legs to either side, the boys sprawl, their eyes glued to the luminous screen, watching two little pigs go about their daily business. In the world of Peppa Pig all things are good. The grown-up pigs are silly and kind. They never get angry with their pig children. The children have dinosaurs and stuffed bears and go to a nursery full of other animals, where they play musical instruments and ride bicycles. Because of their parents' genial disposition, the little pigs are rarely discontent. Their problems, when and if they have them, are always manageable. They do not have post-traumatic stress disorder. My sons like the little pigs a lot. I like the pigs too, mostly due to the fact that the mother pig works from home. The twins compare me frequently to the mother pig, who writes at her computer. 'Mummy!' they shout, if they see me at my desk. 'Tap! Tap! Tap!' And then, gloriously: 'Like Mummy Pig!' It is a joke between them. As I sit with my sons, I think of what Grace had asked when I first told her of my memories: 'Can you do something nice, for the rest of your day?' This is nice. Watching the pigs with my children is nice. They sit on either side of me, nuzzling my arms.

TIME-LINING

I have been told that there are two human responses to the perception of chaos: naming and violence. When the chaos is simply the unknown, the naming can be accomplished effortlessly – a new species, star, formula, equation, prognosis. There is also mapping, charting, or devising proper nouns for unnamed or stripped-of-names geography, landscape or population. When chaos resists, either by reforming itself or rebelling against imposed order, violence is understood to be the most frequent response and the most rational when confronting the unknown, the catastrophic, the wild, wanton, or incorrigible. Rational responses may be censure; incarceration in holding camps, prisons; or death, singly or in war. There is, however, a third response to chaos, which I have not heard about, which is stillness. Such stillness can be passivity and dumbfoundedness; it can be paralytic fear. But it can also be art.

Toni Morrison

As the leaves on the chestnut trees began to burnish, Grace announced that she had arranged a birth debrief at my birth hospital, which would allow me to go over my birth notes with a midwife. She warned me that the research was conflicted in regard to whether these sessions help relieve trauma in birth parents or exacerbate it. Some parents, she said, struggling with birth trauma (mothers, fathers and primary carers alike), may find the hospital setting provided for debriefs distressing and re-traumatising. If the people handling these birth debriefs are not trained in trauma, it is possible that they may inadvertently use language that is upsetting for birth survivors with PTSD.

'Still,' Grace said, 'the debrief may prove therapeutic for you.'

I recalled, then, a steely February day, when I had gone for a walk to the park with Callum. I had wanted, I told Grace, to visit my favourite bench, overlooking an avenue of London plane trees. It took a long time to get there. I lumbered slowly, a brace supporting my belly, as Callum held my arm, worried by my breathlessness. That weekend I'd lost my mucus plug, and had packed my hospital bag and been to see a doctor, who had warned me that the arrival of the twins was imminent, and that my heart was increasingly strained. 'They will come,' a nurse had said, 'any day now.' When we reached the bench, we sat down. Callum told me that he'd booked a table for dinner that evening at a restaurant in town. I asked him to cancel it. All I wanted was to sit here beside him, a moon-faced woman wrapped in a pale scarf, and look at the snow. I confessed that I was frightened, that I did not know what was coming, and that before entering the hospital and meeting our sons, I wanted to remember this, this being here together with him, sitting on the bench, looking out at the quiet snow and the quiet fields and the quiet trees.

I was careful, as we walked home, to avoid slipping on the ice, and it was then that I felt it: the force racing through my body. At home, I sat on the sofa, using an app to count contractions. Callum rang the maternity team at the hospital, who ordered us to come at once to the Antenatal Day Unit, on the seventh floor of the hospital south of the river. Squirting jelly onto Dopplers, the midwives told us that I was in the early stages of labour. They used a machine to count contractions. *One. Two. Three.* I watched as the midwives went hunting for the twins' hearts, searching along the skin of my belly. The midwives struggled with multiples. They could not, for a long time, find Baby B's heart and as the terror engulfed my body, still they could not find my baby's heart. 'Please don't worry,' one of them said, squeezing my hand, and went to ask a colleague. Some midwives have a dowser's gift. One such was summoned: older, wiser, stiller than the rest, she stood to attention above me, listening. Moving the Doppler subtly across my belly, hunting, until, yes, at last, a second galloping rhythm began, and the relief on her face was palpable. I was monitored, prone, with Callum hovering at my side, as the contractions ebbed and flowed. The midwives reassured me that there were two incubators available at this hospital, which was lucky because sometimes pre-term twins must go to separate NICUs at birth. Soon, afternoon turned to dusk, and the midwives sent my husband home. They told me that they would call him later, when I began to dilate. Callum said goodbye, promising to come back as soon as there was any news. I was wheeled in my bed, down the corridor, and told to rest, and await the progression of labour.

I entered a ward occupied by other women. The first watched a film, headphones plugged into her iPad, with the calm focus of a soldier. She did not acknowledge my existence or say hello and I did not feel, at this point, much like introducing myself either because at the exact moment of my arrival, a second visibly pregnant woman was screaming out in agony. I heard a doctor delivering bad news – that the baby will not live, that the labour came too early – and the woman was weeping now, and also labouring, and she screamed with each contraction. Curtains were drawn then, around my own bed, but they could not block it out: the bone-chilling power of the woman's grief. I too began to cry. As a midwife checked on my own contractions, the curtains once again parted and I saw the miscarrying woman being strapped to a gurney, reaching out to her husband, tears pouring down her cheeks. As soon as I witnessed this, she was gone, swept out of the room in a blur. For a long time afterwards, I did not move. I cried a bit in bed, then heaved myself out of bed in my hospital gown and cried as I brushed my teeth. I cried as I waddled back to bed, glancing again at the woman plugged into her iPad, her face illuminated by the flickering screen. A cleaner changed the miscarrying woman's bloodied sheets, crumpling them into a large blue bag. I watched her spray down the bare plastic bed and wipe it dry.

The cleaner was focused and methodical, and like the woman on the iPad, remained, as far as I could tell, entirely unmoved.

While I got into my pyjamas, another pregnant woman took the freshly made bed vacated by the miscarrying mother. The anxiety radiating off this woman was palpable. She could not feel her baby moving and was absolutely terrified. She repeated this to everyone who came to check on her, and I grew equally terrified on her behalf. Eventually she was taken away for a scan. She returned jubilant. The baby was alive, and not only alive, soon to make its arrival in this world. That night, the sounds of the labouring woman in the bed across from mine were warm and earthy and round.

At midnight a midwife came to see me. She told me I would give birth soon and injected me with a steroid shot, to ready my babies' pre-term lungs for arrival. She warned me it would be painful, but I did not feel much of anything. After this, I could not sleep. I lay very still. At three in the morning, the third labouring woman vanished like the miscarrying woman to the birthing suites, and I got out of bed for a wander. I waddled down the empty, darkened hall of the Antenatal Day Unit, looking for the common area. When I found it, I made myself a cup of tea in the dark, standing at the window, looking at the lights of the city. I called my mother, then, in California, worried about my father's biopsy.

'Hello,' I said, 'how are you?'

The steam from my teacup smudged up the window, and as my mother spoke, the mysterious force inside my body stopped. The contractions whipping round my belly ebbed and flowed, gradually petering out to nothing.

The next morning, I lumbered to the communal bathroom and brushed my teeth again. As I exited the bathroom, the silent pregnant woman plugged into her iPad took out her ear buds and said hello. She had observed my pattern of behaviour and liked me, she said, because I was quiet. 'Not many people around here are quiet.' She invited me to eat breakfast with her. The woman had heard from the midwives that I was carrying twins. So was she, she said, although she had been bleeding now for weeks. 'That's why I'm here,' she said. She had been living in this shared room for a month, bleeding intermittently, and must stay here, day and night, until she gave birth. That could take weeks, she said, though she hoped for months – while living here wasn't particularly pleasant, it was worth it. The midwives and nurses were kind and attentive, and she'd found a little routine to pass the time. She wore compression socks every day, and had scans, and watched movies on her iPad and read books. She moved very little – and this was working – she recommended not moving as a technique for me. She moved, she said, only enough to get the blood flowing round her body and avoid clots. Her husband visited once a day to see her, after work, and occasionally, so did friends.

Only one thing bothered her: she was sick – sick to death – of the food. On the basis of the food, she did not know how she'd get through the next few weeks, but she'd do any-thing – anything – for her babies. What she went through, before coming here, was harrowing. Here, at least, help is at hand, and it's a waiting game, isn't it, after all?

She was in a particularly good mood today because she recently crossed a magic gestational line for pre-term deliveries: her babies had reached two pounds in weight and buoyed by this achievement, she hoped to push on, keeping them inside a few weeks longer. She saw them regularly on the ultrasound and their aliveness filled her with hope – before them she suffered multiple miscarriages – but 'when they come now,' she said, 'they'll have a fighting chance. Much better than before.'

I told her that I too had suffered miscarriages, that this was my third pregnancy. I told her that her stoicism impressed me, and she batted this away with her hand.

'You get by,' she said.

I wondered, privately – I did not ask her – how many women she had witnessed lose their baby in the bed beside her and how many more she'd witness over the weeks before her own were born.

She told me that I was lucky. 'You're almost thirty-five weeks,' she said, knowledgeably. She'd done her research and was confident that thirty-five weeks was good for pre-term babies. 'No matter what happens now, they'll be all right; every day is a victory.'

As she said this she glanced meaningfully in the direction of the bereaved woman's husband, the man we had seen weeping with his miscarrying wife, eating his breakfast alone.

I did not go into labour that afternoon. When I left the ward, the woman carrying twins took off her headphones. She sat up. She said goodbye from her bed. 'Good luck,' I said, and she echoed the same back to me, but I could feel a distance growing between us: the anxiety in her *good luck*, the hint of sadness. I watched as she returned to her prone position, lying on her side, in the ubiquitous hospital bed, plugged into her iPad, the glare of the screen illuminating the determination in her face.

At home, I followed the advice of the midwives and the long-suffering mother of twins I met in the ADU: I pursued stillness. My mother-in-law invited me to stay in her spare room. She looked after me there, while my husband was away at work. Her kindness ensured that I did not have to move. I did not leave her house except to the garden, where I sat on a bench wrapped in a blanket, and watched a robin singing in the branches of a bare apple tree. Bed rest for me, unlike the woman at the ADU, was a pleasant experience: my mother-in-law brought cream teas to my room, and kept me company. I watched snow settling from my bedroom window, and wrote on my laptop in bed, a human incubator.

Without explanation, my thirty-six-week scan was cancelled and I was not offered another in its place. I returned to my apartment, thirty-seven weeks pregnant and happy, confident that my twins were safe. At my next hospital appointment I was told that my obstetrician had scheduled me for an induction. My younger brother had come to stay in London after the fire in California, and moved into my apartment to look after me. He said often, watching me shuffle breathlessly around, taking my arm as I heaved my way upstairs, that he felt worried but could not put his finger on why. Wanting labour to start now, I moved a bit, sat down, moved again. I loaded and unloaded the dishwasher. I attempted to jump, but could not get my feet off the floor. I read advice online on how to bring on labour naturally:

I ate spicy curries, drank vast quantities of red raspberry leaf tea, saw an acupuncturist, downed cod liver oil. The babies did not budge. The hospital called on the day of my scheduled induction, to say, sorry no, we're overflowing with expectant mothers, there's no room at the inn. My brother was outraged on my behalf. I was told I would have to wait a number of days for a slot to open and that I would be called, an hour or two before. My brother burst out, 'Is that safe?'

Was anything safe?

At my last scan, at thirty-four weeks, Baby B was transverse, and what I read online about delivering transverse babies frightened me. I rang the hospital and asked for a follow-up scan, and a caesarean, but they did not think it necessary. Another day passed and the twins did not budge. The next evening, when the hospital still had not called to say come in, a new fear, specific to multiple gestation, kicked in: I was now approaching the end of the thirty-seventh week. I had read and reread NICE Regulations which stated that all multiples should be born by the end of the thirty-seventh week of gestation, at the latest. I rang again, asking to be assessed by an obstetrician. None was available. I was told that if I wanted to see a doctor, I should go back to the Antenatal Day Unit at the hospital and wait until a doctor on call could consult with me. I went to the hospital at once, with my brother, who left when my husband joined me after work. I waited five hours to see a doctor, reading a novel. I did not mind this, sitting and waiting: patience felt important.

Finally, a young man in scrubs appeared, a doctor, asking tersely: 'What's the matter?'

I said that my induction was scheduled to start two days ago but had been delayed and delayed again by the hospital.

Now I did not know when it would happen.

I said, 'I'm carrying multiples, one of whom is transverse,

and in another day's time, I will reach the end of the thirty-seventh week of gestation.'

I reminded the doctor of the NICE regulation guidelines, which stated clearly that giving birth to multiples at thirty-eight weeks carried higher risks of complications and mortality, and then I challenged him: 'Surely it would be safer to have my babies by scheduled C-section, rather than inducing labour?'

The obstetrician brushed this off: he was not worried.

But was an induction of a transverse twin *really* safe?

'Look,' I said, panicking, 'I haven't had a scan at your hospital since I went into pre-term labour at thirty-four weeks. I am a high-risk mother of multiples and a month has elapsed now, without any ultrasound. I have no idea what's going on inside my body right now: no one at your hospital has any idea of what's going on inside my body. Are you not worried by this? Surely I need a scan? Surely a planned caesarean would be better?'

He looked at me blankly. 'I don't really understand what you want me to do.'

His confusion puzzled me.

Was I not being clear?

I tried harder.

He flicked through my notes. All my anxieties, he said, were unfounded.

'I don't see a problem with going ahead with your induction. No need, in my opinion, to schedule a C-section. There aren't slots available.'

But was this safe?

The doctor, who was handsome and fit, glanced at his watch, irritated now. 'Birth is safe,' he snapped. 'It's a natural process, not a disease, and having an induction is safer than having a caesarean.' He talked at a clip, in his scrubs, blood

341

on his apron: 'I really don't have time to get into the details of your decision but, at this point, stick with the induction. You're fine. You'll be fine.' He assured me that the pain in my belly was a normal variant of multiple gestation: 'You've done a good job,' he said, 'getting this far.

'Besides,' he added, pointing to my stomach, 'anything happens, we'll be right in there. Bang!' He mimicked an explosion with his hands. 'Emergency caesareans, they're our A-bomb, our secret weapon. Any problem? We go nuclear.'

People never speak of a mother's intelligence, *as if that would diminish her affectivity, distance her as a mother. But intelligence is everything that permits us to live superlatively with another person.*

Roland Barthes, 15 April 1977

'No one who hurt you,' Grace said, 'has ever had to face the consequences of their actions. It is vital,' she said, 'when it comes to your birth experience, that you demand to know exactly what happened to you, that you ask *why*.' Grace arranged the debrief for mid-October. Leading up to this, Grace asked if I would be comfortable tackling the numbness and amnesia I felt around my sons' birth experience head-on.

Decades after treatment, the famous hysterical patient 'Fräulein Anna O' (née Bertha Pappenheim), the girl who coined the phrase the *talking cure*, the 'actual founder' (Freud said) 'of the psychoanalytical approach', the incurable patient/ *cause célèbre* whose symptoms included paralysis, hallucinations, bouts of mutism and a phantom pregnancy conceived by her therapist, reflected on her time with the renowned Austrian psychologist Josef Breuer.

O observed: Psychoanalysis, in the hands of the physician, is what confession is in the hands of the Catholic priest; it depends on its user and its use whether it becomes a beneficial tool or a two-edged sword.

I recounted then, how, on the eve of my children's birth, a stranger's fingers inserted a pessary into my cervix, and a mysterious switch went off in my body and I was gone. This absence, Grace said, was very likely the beginning of an episode of dissociation, stemming from denial of traumatic events. The force of denial has surprising physical and neurological effects on the body. In some cases – like my own – the dissociating person enters such an extreme state of numbness that they lose all sensation of pain. As I laboured, I drifted high above my husband and came back down only briefly to ask the midwife what contractions felt like. She responded kindly that for everyone the sensations are different, unique to their own body. She asked me if I was experiencing pain and I said no. I told her the truth: that I was on a train, hurtling forward, and something powerful was happening within me, something powerful and out of control – but my mind floated high above it and so I felt something and also nothing. I told her I believed I was having contractions.

'Labouring women do not feel something and also nothing,' the midwife said. She told me that when women entered labour they felt powerful waves, of tension, and release, of pain.

She put her hands on my back, she held me, she soothed me.

'We are here to help,' she said, 'we are here to guide you through it, to support you, to usher your babies into this world.'

Labouring women, they scream, they moan, they hyperventilate, they rock from side to side, they ask for relief. As I was doing none of these things, she encouraged me to take a bath.

I entered the water, alone, in the little bathroom adjacent to the ward, and my bowels opened. I relieved myself entirely and began to vomit. It was hard to scramble, up, out of the bath, it was hard to clean everything, I felt embarrassed, I felt sick, I threw up again and again, as I cleaned, and in the terror, in the pain, my heart shattered.

Terror, silence, numbness, gone.

Callum helped me back onto the bed as my waters broke. The midwife came back to my bed, shocked. 'You are five centimetres dilated,' she said. 'It's only been two hours since the pessary went in. You're going have these babies soon,' she said, 'you're going to have these babies fast.' I was given a mandatory epidural, a requirement for all vaginal multiples deliveries at my birth hospital. I did not have any choice in this matter. The midwife and anaesthetist asked me to sit still, stay still. So I sat very still. 'Can you feel anything?' they asked. No, first, then: 'Yes,' I said. 'Yes. Yes, I do.' They pulled the needle out, plunged it in again. I absented myself, I obeyed. I accepted everything in this place. I never shouted, never screamed. *She is quiet, she is still, she is brave, she is strong,* the midwives said. 'Both babies,' they told me, as the first began to crown, 'they are back to back, spine to spine, they are the wrong way round.' A moving bed. A folder, thrust in front of me. Pen. Paper. A dotted line. 'Sign here.' Sign what? Give consent to what? I signed. When women asked me to push, I pushed.

When women asked me to breathe, I breathed. I asked my husband, writing this, if I was silent during their birth also, and he said, 'Yes, come to think of it, you did not make a sound.'

I cannot remember, clearly, precisely what happened after my children's exodus, try and try as I might. When it is over, all I have is an image of a masked, unbreathing baby flying out of the room, and another child lifted crying from my chest, and then the bleeding and the coming and the going, the pulling and the tugging, surrounded yet alone in the little room. I try, with Grace's help, to excavate more, to catch fragments. Little glimmers of hope. Little shards of understanding. I cast myself as a detective. Truth seeker. Someone, I remembered, knocked at the door. 'The high-dependency unit is full.' My consultant obstetrician, next, a woman who did not deliver the babies but arranged my induction, appeared surreally from the sidelines, like an umpire or a standing judge. She shook my hand. 'You were magnificent.' What? I stared at her. A little crowd, then. Clapping. People clapping. Everyone clapping. Some time later, a small, harried face, nervous, uniformed. 'Could you tell me what happened? We don't have,' the woman said, 'any of your notes.' There it goes again: the flickering.

As I sat cross-legged on a blanket, in the park, the babies, for the first time, assumed a position on each of my thighs. They drank as wild animals drink, standing upright, kneading my breasts, burrowing into my skin, tugging at a nipple, gumming the teat, pulling the milk down; I supported their chubby bodies with my hands, holding them in place. I believe the language of rape within maternal mental health has been established largely on the basis of silence. A silence that buries and denies, and excises and obscures, in order to survive. I have not tried to write a medical history of the intersection of sexual assault and assault in childbirth, but rather excavate that silence, within the archaeology of my own life.

When the twins were seven months old, my little family and I flew home to California, where home as I knew it had disappeared. My dad picked us up from the airport in Los Angeles, warning us that it would take a little longer than usual, three or four hours, to drive home due to traffic. We landed during the Woolsey Fire of November 2018, a blaze that ravaged the Malibu coastline north of Los Angeles. My father was not at all perturbed by this. The twins slept soundly in the back of the car, along with my husband, and my father suggested I do the same, but how could I sleep? 'Dad,' I said, 'look.' We looked out, beyond the highway, and saw flames shooting up the ridgeline like comets. I asked my father if this is how the Thomas Fire had been, and he said, yes, and then no, that inferno last year was worse. Much worse. Clouds of ash had filled the air and they had to wear masks to breathe and the sky had turned a horrible, violent red that lasted for days and days and days. 'It was,' he mused, 'like an apocalypse.'

The next day, Callum and I made the solemn pilgrimage to the place where the house had been. A storm had rolled in that morning from the high mountains and my parents did not want to come, claiming to be busy. I drove us up the winding Dennison Grade, with our seven-month-old sons sleeping in the back. Around each bend I said stupidly to Callum: 'That's gone.' But because Callum had not grown up here, because he had not memorised the exact position of the structures that made up the subtle landscape of my childhood – the bright roofs among scrub oaks, the seventies wood houses, perched on ridgelines – because he had not been to spiritual teachings at the Ojai Foundation (destroyed in the flames) or walked in the gardens of Meditation Mount (burned at its perimeter, but survived) holding a battered copy of the Indian philosopher Jiddu Krishnamurti's journal, which contains the best description of my home I had ever read, Callum struggled to make sense of my losses, for he could not recall how things were. Later, shaken by absence, seeking confirmation that what I remembered was true, I would return to *Krishnamurti's Journal*, to the forty-first entry, written on 8 April 1975:

In this part of the world it doesn't rain much, about fifteen to twenty inches a year, and these rains are most welcome for it doesn't rain for the rest of the year. There is snow then on the mountains and during summer and

autumn they are bare, sunburnt, rocky and forbidding;
only in the spring are they mellow and welcoming. There
used to be bear, deer, bob cat, quail and any number of
rattlers. But now they are disappearing; the dreaded man
is encroaching. It had rained for some time now and the
valley was green, the orange trees bore fruit and flower.
It is a beautiful valley, quiet away from the village, and
you heard the mourning dove. The air was slowly being
filled with the scent of orange blossoms and in a few days
it would be overpowering, with the warm sun and wind-
less days. It was a valley wholly surrounded by hills and
mountains; beyond the hills was the sea and beyond the
mountains, desert. In the summer it would be unbeara-
bly hot but there was always beauty here, far from the
maddening crowd and their cities. And at night there
would be extraordinary silence, rich and penetrating. The
cultivated meditation is a sacrilege to beauty, and every
leaf and branch spoke of the joy of beauty and the tall
dark cypress was silent with it; the gnarled old pepper
tree flowed with it.

It was cloudy when we drove up the Highway 126, on
that particular November morning, but it was not green.
The air was not full of the scent of orange blossoms. The
scrub oaks had burned to black stumps, the carcasses of
houses had been cleared, and in their place, I found scars
in the wilderness – flat patches of furrowed earth. To the
north, looking at the great Los Padres National Forest, the
mountains, as far as the eye could see, were naked. Stripped
bare of any foliage, they looked toothy and ashen, full of
undiscovered features: great rocks and boulders, strangers to
my childhood memories, seams of ugly yellow earth. When
I looked down into the valley I grew up in, I saw a village

ringed by devastation. The orange trees had survived, and so too had the town within, but the foothills? The foothills had burned beyond recognition and the animals had vanished. I'd heard stories from my mother of the creatures who came seeking refuge after the fire, asking humans for help. The bear cub who had to be put down. The silver fox, once a fixture on our hill – the same fox who used to drink water from the horses' trough – came to see my parents when they first returned to the house after the fire, limping. The fur had been singed off his tail, his burned paws were raw and bleeding. My parents left food out for him, but he died. As for the deer, who my mother both loved and hated because they ate the rose bushes, they had not been seen by any member of the family for months. I parked the car and got out at my parents' property – what they called The Land – and I looked at the five black stumps of the cypress trees that I had dreamed of in hospital. The babies were still sleeping, so Callum and I left them in the car, with the doors open, and walked gingerly forward, holding hands.

Every leaf and branch spoke of the joy of beauty and the tall dark cypress was silent with it . . .

'It's gone,' I said to Callum standing in the place the kitchen had been, looking out over the scorched earth.

'It's really gone.'

The clouds joined together, the flood fell down on the mountains.

The babies woke.

Walking back, with Callum, through the rain, towards my crying children, I studied the atomised pieces of my mother's crockery, pummelled into earth, and thought, *This is it: this is what the numbness looks like.* This is what it does to your mind, to your body, to your sense of self. Fragments it. Fire is an incomplete act of erasure. A house disappears, and yet the shape of it remains hanging in the air, such that you can almost see it. In birth, we too contain multitudes: past, present, future selves, and if the labour of coming into motherhood is too excruciating, too unbearably eviscerating, we can be left in ruins.

In *The Body Keeps the Score*, Bessel van der Kolk's seminal work on Trauma, he wryly observes that therapists (and perhaps also writers) 'have an undying faith in the capacity of talk to resolve trauma'. Kolk goes on to explain that this 'confidence dates back to 1893 when Freud (and his mentor, Breuer) wrote that trauma "immediately and permanently disappeared when we had succeeded in bringing clearly to light the memory of the event by which it was provoked and in arousing its accompanying affect, and when the patient had described that event in the greatest possible detail and had put the affect into words."'

'Unfortunately,' Kolk continues, 'it's not so simple: traumatic events are almost impossible to put into words.'

The paradox of wordlessness, within the wordfulness of writing, is manifest.

I had written my first novel long before becoming a mother, within trauma, about trauma, without the tools or the understanding or the words to control or process it. I had perpetuated violent myths. Committed violent acts. I had severed tongues, dismembered bodies. I wrote in broken patterns, repeated ellipses. I deliberately assaulted my protagonist. I took her right up to the edge of dying, heightened, hysterical, unreal. She escaped. But when it came to the point of continuing her story, I could not progress her narrative forward. I did not know how to: I did not know how to authentically progress a woman's story forward, in the wake of assault. I did not know how to resolve her anger, her depression, her trauma and bereavement, because I had not resolved those things within myself. The same frustrations, the same corrosive anger, came to haunt me after birth. Things had been done to me I could not erase, could not change.

I learned, from Grace, as I pieced birth memories back together, that mothers (or birth partners) who dissociate during labour or birth are more likely to develop PTSD postnatally than those who do not. This is why, she said, it is so important for midwives and obstetricians to have additional training in trauma, so that they can help identify when a birthing mother or birth partner may have entered a dissociative state. Once a mother has dissociated, she may struggle to connect with her babies during her birth experience and may also struggle to remember what happened during the episode of dissociation.

After birth, I asked questions. I asked everyone I could. I asked, 'What happened to me in that room?' The midwives looked at the screens in their hands and the little printed notes on the side of my bed and said: 'Natural labour, normal vaginal delivery, thirty-six weeks' gestation, manual removal of placenta, ragged membranes, forceps and ventouse, second-degree tear, episiotomy, blood loss,' And then weirdly, surreally: 'No complications.'

No complications? 'Please,' I say. 'Your notes are wrong. I gave birth at thirty-eight weeks. I had an induction. Please. I had complications. I must have had complications. Something is missing. Something hurts, deep inside me.'

The system says: No, no, no, nothing missing. Nothing missing. But I can feel it. 'No,' the midwives reply, reading their notes. Each time they come to my bed, I ask them. Your pain is normal. It is from your uterus contracting. It is from the catheter. It is from the stitches. 'Please,' I say. 'This pain is different. Please. Listen. This is important. Please. I need blood.' 'According to our notes, you do not need blood.' I lost a lot of blood. Please. I saw blood. Please. There were bags of blood. Bowls of blood. Please. I cannot walk. I cannot move. Please. I am in pain. Please. My husband is not here. He is with my son in NICU. Please, I have two babies. Please. I cannot wash myself. Please. I have collapsed in the bathroom. I have hit my head on the ceramic. Please. I am pressing this button for a reason. Please. Listen. Please. I am not trying to be difficult. Please. Tell me. Something happened in that room. Something that has a name.

'After that,' I said to Grace, 'I don't know.'

In the last month of therapy, Grace journeyed into the fog that had descended at birth, armed with pen and paper. She scribbled down notes, made connections. She worked methodically. Analysing my recollections of birth, examining things that troubled me. 'Time-lining', as she put it, rearranging disjointed fragments, putting them into chronological order, marking it out in thin, red ink. She encouraged me to do the same.

But I did not feel like writing and so laid a blanket out, beneath the auburn trees, and helped the boys with tummy time. They played awhile, kicking their legs, pushing up on chubby forearms. Shifting their weight backwards and forwards, teaching themselves to crawl. Look at the bugs, the bugs in the grass. Look at the dry leaves. Look at the spiked green envelopes of fresh chestnuts. They reached out for these things, hitching themselves forward, they tugged and clutched at the earth, pulling fistfuls towards their mouths. I cleaned their fingers, tutting. I tickled their feet, their cherubim folds. They laughed raucous baby belly laughs, hiccuping little crescendos of song. I found them so beautiful. 'Hello,' I said. 'Hello.' They cooed and giggled and fidgeted and stopped, suddenly, transfixed again by something new, lying on their backs, staring. I mirrored them, laying down on the earth, curling my body around theirs, holding their little mud-stained fingers. 'Look,' I said, pointing. Together we looked at the leaves on the trees. 'Look at the light.'

I decided, then, to begin my own time-lining.

1847. Birth of Fanny Longfellow, wife of the prominent American poet. Her mother famously takes ether in labour. Six years later, Queen Victoria, following the advice of her physicians, popularises the use of chloroform in childbirth.

1896. Freud, publishing *The Aetiology of Hysteria*, puts forward the thesis:

> *that at the bottom of every case of hysteria there are one or more occurrences of premature sexual experience, occurrences which belong to the earliest years of childhood, but which can be reproduced through the work of psycho-analysis in spite of the intervening decades. I believe that this is an important finding, the discovery of a caput Nili in neuropathology.*

Caput Nili, from the Latin, literally *the head of the Nile*, as in searching for the source of the river. Used metaphorically by Romans to refer to a problem that appeared unsolvable. Freud's finding that the root of hysteria lay in childhood experiences of sexual abuse (later known as Seduction Theory) was met with horror in Vienna. He wrote of the fallout in a letter to a friend: '*I am as isolated as you could wish me to be: the word has been given out to abandon me, and a void is forming around me*'.

1917. Young officer and pacifist Siegfried Sassoon, having famously denounced the war, arrives at Craiglockhart War Hospital in Scotland, battling something he calls 'the unspeakable tragedy of shellshock'. At Craiglockhart, Sassoon enters into the care of Rivers, an enigmatic army doctor, who listens, with wry conviviality, while Sassoon talks. During his rehabilitation, Sassoon catalogues the nuances of a mental disorder afflicting soldiers plagued by recollection of war. 'Not then was their evil hour,' Sassoon would later write, 'but now; now, in the sweating suffocation of nightmare, in paralysis of limbs, in the stammering of dislocated speech'. When Sassoon finishes his treatment with Rivers, he is sent, again, to the Front, where a British soldier accidentally wounds Sassoon, shooting Sassoon in the head, after mistaking him for a German. Sassoon, surviving this, will refashion his therapeutic dialogue with Rivers into George Sherston's fictionalised memoirs.

Sassoon is buried in the West Country. I have stood at his graveside midwinter, holding my sons' hands, and walked down the spectral avenue of yew to soft, snow-covered fields. Trudging through the snow, I have thought of Grace's little room, not unlike Rivers's, and how Sherston, returning to the Font, pulling Rivers's door shut for the last time, had 'left behind someone who had helped and understood me more than anyone I had ever known'. I am not the first to draw a parallel between birth trauma and shellshock. In Jacqueline Rose's erudite analysis of Euripides, she highlights a Graeco-Roman 'analogy between parturition and the injuries of war', citing Medea's gauntlet on motherhood:

> They, men, allege that we enjoy a life
> secure from danger safe at home,
> while they confront the thrusting spears of war.
> I would rather join
> the battle rank of shields three times
> than undergo birth's labour once.

1926. American psychologists Edward A. Strecker and Franklin G. Ebaugh, in their study *Psychoses occurring during the puerperium*, argue emphatically that postpartum depression has no relation to pregnancy, childbirth or the lactation period: this was all conjecture. Postpartum depression was a subcategory mood disorder at best indistinct from other psychiatric illness. They call on American psychiatrists to eliminate the term from their vocabulary. Following their advice, the American Psychiatric Association and American Medical Association removed postpartum depression from their diagnostic manuals.

1929. Zilboorg, who treated Gershwin and examined Hemingway, believes that depressed mothers rejected their babies as a means of fleeing from reality. He attributes postpartum depression to pre-pregnancy frigid personalities. Also: repressed homosexual urges, unresolved Oedipal longings, and anal-regressive resultant father identification. Whatever that means.

1962. The American doctor and esteemed psychiatrist James Hamilton publishes *Postpartum Psychiatric Problems.* Inspired by the French psychologist Marcé, who had studied cases of Puerperal Insanity at Salpêtrière in the 1850s, Hamilton focuses his research around biological and hormonal changes in the postpartum body. Hamilton remarks that the onset of most postpartum disturbances were insidious and sudden. After birth, he notes, the mother entering psychosis often experienced a lucid interval, before being overwhelmed by confusion or delirium. These changes in mood, Hamilton believed, like Marcé and the Hippocratic authors before him, were not phantoms of the mind, but *somatic*, caused by changes rooted in the body.

1964. Ralph S. Paffenbarger, Jr., searching for a cause of mental illnesses related to childbearing, publishes *Epidemiological Aspects of Parapartum Mental Illness*, a large study funded by a research grant from the National Heart Institute and US Public Health Service. Summarising his findings, Paffenbarger observes that postpartum mental illness patients 'had shorter gestation periods, stormier pregnancies, more dystocia, and infants of lighter birth weight and higher perinatal mortality'. His research also suggests that post partum 'disturbances' were potentially somatic in origin, related to endocrine imbalance in the body.

1969. Boston, Massachusetts. Wendy Sanford, mother, wife, goes to the doctor complaining of a problem: she can't stop crying while her baby naps. On a panel in 2014, hosted by the Gender and Sexualities Program at Boston University, Wendy would recall how, as a twenty-six-year-old mother in 1969, she had tried:

> *speaking to my ob/gyn about how I was feeling. Across the expanse of his desk, I told him how I sank to the living room floor and cried while my baby napped, pressing my cheek against the carpet, how I felt like I was falling apart. The doctor laid a hand on mine. 'Don't want too much,' he said, patting. 'This is what I like to tell my new mothers: Get out to a library once in a while to keep your mind going and your spirits up, but be satisfied.'*

A while later, Wendy got a call from a friend, who was setting up an informal course on Women's Health in an MIT lounge. Wendy initially declined; she had a nine-month-old baby and she was tired. 'I didn't go the first week,' Wendy said, but when the next session rolled around, a friend came to pick Wendy up in a car. Wendy found herself in a crowded MIT lounge, where a woman was giving an animated lecture on masturbation using a life-size diagram. After the talk, the crowd broke into smaller classrooms for more intimate discussions. The conversation in Wendy's group ranged from orgasm to breastfeeding. Suddenly, one of the young women, who was also mothering a newborn, confessed that for months she had felt awful – not physically awful, but emotionally. 'What is it?' Wendy had asked, finally breaking her silence, 'what did you do?' The woman said that she had something called Postpartum Depression. Wendy felt stunned:

What I had been feeling had a name. It was a real phenomenon, with physical and societal causes, and it wasn't my fault. The nuclear family could be a lonely place for mothers, the women said. What I experienced as I blotched the yellow living room rug with tears while my baby napped was part of a societal picture that I could learn about—that perhaps, with others, I could change. I felt a glimmer of elation, as if someone had lifted the flap of a heavy tarp that had settled on me, letting in light, a gust of air.

Wendy would go on to co-author *Our Bodies, Ourselves* in 1971, joining a collective of Boston women, many of whom were mothers, who pioneered the Women's Health Movement. A radical, underground success, *Our Bodies, Ourselves* (which began life as a revolutionary course booklet on stapled newsprint) would become a word of mouth hit, selling like hot cakes.

1977. Ian Brockington, a forty-two-year-old senior lecturer at Manchester, with a growing interest in the psychiatry of motherhood and disordered mother–infant bonding, writes to the American clinician James Hamilton (of *Postpartum Psychiatric Problems* fame) regarding a mother struggling with a bonding disorder (a condition then described by Brockington as '*terra incognita*'). Following his conversation with Hamilton, Brockington organises a meeting with Ramesh 'Channi' Kumar, professor of perinatal psychiatry at the Institute of Psychiatry, King's College London, whose focus was on the importance of mother–baby bonding and breastfeeding, and Merton Sandler, freemason, professor in chemical biology, and pioneer in biological psychology, whose original work in the field led to the development of antidepressants in 1959. This conversation, as per Brockington, 'stimulated British interest in puerperal mental health', and led to the publication of *Mental Illness in Pregnancy and the Puerperium*, through Oxford University Press in 1978.

1980. Buoyed by the enthusiastic reception of his research, Ian Brockington arranges an international conference of 150 delegates on perinatal mental health, to which he invites American expert James Hamilton. Decades later, Brockington recalled:

Someone compared James Hamilton to John the Baptist, and Merton raised the roof by saying that his quotations from Marcé were like the Pope's Christmas message. I could be wrong, but I think it was James Hamilton who introduced Marcé's writings to us. He brought both his major works to show us. Of course he read the French with a wonderful American accent.

On the eve of the conference, Brockington hosts a reception at his house in Manchester, for thirty speakers, at which he serves lobster salad. A second soirée takes place at the Manchester Art Gallery. Following the extravaganza, Brockington and his wife host a private dinner party attended by the three American stars of the conference, Jim Hamilton, Ralph Paffenbarger, Jr., and George Winokur, and two Britons, Channi Kumar, and Robert Kendell, all experts in the field. Over dinner, the men lay the foundations of the International Marcé Society for Perinatal Mental Health (still in existence today). Ian Brockington would be its first president, Channi Kumar its second.

1981. Dr Channi Kumar participates in the creation of a mother-baby unit at Maudsley Hospital in London, where he carries out several research projects. He aims to treat postpartum mental illness while supporting mothers who wish to continue to breastfeed. His work looks closely at maternal filicide under psychosis. Previous to Kumar's findings, mothers in the United Kingdom were routinely separated from their children during treatment for postpartum depression and psychosis, the most severe cases requiring institutionalisation in mental health facilities. Strengthening the mother–child bond during this period was paramount: crucial, Kumar believed, in recovery.

2001. American clinical practitioner and certified nurse midwife Cheryl Tatano Beck (having devoted fifteen years of her life to the study of postnatal depression) travels to New Zealand, to give a keynote address on perinatal anxiety disorders at the Australasian Marcé Society Biennial Scientific meeting in Christchurch. At that time, she writes:

> *I [had come] across a small number of studies on an anxiety disorder I had not heard of – PTSD due to childbirth. Of course, I knew about PTSD, but had never connected this anxiety disorder to women as a result of their giving birth.*

After Beck delivers her talk, a second woman approaches the podium: Sue Watson, a mother who suffered PTSD following birth, and had gone on to found a charitable trust in New Zealand called Trauma and Birth Stress. It was, Beck recalls, as if the world stood still: 'You could have heard a pin drop.'

2004. Three years later, working with Sue Watson, Cheryl Tatano Beck publishes a qualitative study of birth trauma in forty women, titled *Birth Trauma: In the eye of the beholder.*

'What became apparent,' Beck observes, was that the women who felt traumatised by birth, had been 'systematically stripped of protective layers of caring'.

Beck defines Birth Trauma as:

An event occurring during the labor and delivery process that involves actual or threatened serious injury or death to the mother and her infant. The birthing woman experiences intense fear, helplessness, loss of control, and horror.

'I felt like a piece of meat on the bed. After I was afraid to look at myself in the mirror. I was afraid to look at myself in the eyes,' one mother recounted in the study. 'I felt like my soul had died.'

Beck has subsequently revised that definition, to include 'an event occurring during labor or delivery where the woman perceives that she is stripped of her dignity'.

2006. Sheila Kitzinger, *Birth Crisis*. Routledge Press.

The experiences of women who have been sexually abused represent in microcosm those of all women who feel degraded and abused by what is done to them in pregnancy and childbirth. When birth is conducted with no personal consideration and respect, when management is crude and insensitive, it is itself a form of sexual abuse.

2008. M. Sperlich and J. S. Seng publish *Survivor Moms: Women's stories of birthing, mothering and healing after sexual abuse.* Sperlich and Seng find (anecdotally) that 'survivors of sexual abuse struggle to trust in their bodies during childbirth', because of 'the violation of their bodies' in their past.

2013. Cheryl Tatano Beck, circling round *Traumatic Childbirth*, writing of the latest research into postpartum PTSD, seeks hope in the ashes. She, like Sperlich and Seng, warns that birth can be a triggering experience for abuse survivors. Reviewing risk factors for developing PTSD post-partum, Beck emphasises that 're-traumatization taking place at one of the important events in a woman's life increases the negative power of this trauma. If, however,' she concludes, 'a woman feels she has received caring, competent support from labour and delivery staff and she has successfully met the challenges of birthing her infant, she can experience increased empowerment.' Beck builds on evidence gathered by American doula Penny Simpkin and psychotherapist and social worker Phyllis Klaus, in their collaboration, *When Survivors Give Birth,* which suggests that phrases like 'trust your body' and 'do what your body tells you to do' can bring up intensely negative feelings in survivors of childhood sexual abuse during labour. So, too, commands from obstetricians and nurses like 'open your legs' or 'relax and it won't hurt as much'. Among survivors with perinatal mood disorders, Simpkin and Klaus note, postpartum PTSD 'deserves special mention since it is frequently linked with a history of sexual abuse', often emerging in association with a specific trauma: 'either the recent birth,' Simpkin and Klaus write, 'or memories from the past that were triggered during birth'.

2016. Pavan Amara, herself the survivor of rape, founds The My Body Back Maternity Clinic at St Bartholomew's, in London, the first designated maternity clinic for rape survivors worldwide. Amara, working with the NHS, pioneers a 'different birthing pathway' to ensure that the patients at the maternity clinic – pregnant rape survivors – 'receive tailored, sensitive care'. Coinciding with the clinic's opening, Amara writes an article for the *Independent*, titled 'Pregnancy and Birth can be dangerously traumatic for Rape Victims. Now I've found a way to help'. In her article, Amara shares the case-history of one of her patients – alias 'Sarah' – who violently recalled assault in birth.

> *Last year I met a woman who told me that, apart from the day she was raped, giving birth to her child was the most traumatic day of her life. Throughout labour and her baby son's first few hours of life, images of her rapist's face and of the rape itself continuously flashed through her mind. With vaginal examinations being carried out, contractions forcing her out of control of her own body, and strangers constantly touching her without her consent, she began remembering and reliving the rape that she thought she had left behind many years before. If that was hard for you to read, imagine how hard it is to endure. For those first, crucial, hours of her child's life she couldn't bond with him because she was too busy trying to keep herself sane.*

I find Amara's article, googling search terms after therapy with Grace, and feel the same radical bolt of self-recognition that Wendy Sanford described in 1969: *What I had been feeling had a name*. If this reliving of rape was so common among survivors, as Amara suggested, surely it could be screened for among women across maternity services? Why didn't it merit broader interest? David J. Morris argues in *The Evil Hours: A Biography of Post-Traumatic Stress Disorder* that the experience of female survivors of sexual trauma remains broadly occluded in Western society, and the study (and treatment) of trauma remains broadly gendered. 'Despite the fact that rape is the most common and most injurious form of trauma,' Morris continues, 'the bulk of PTSD research is directed towards war trauma and veterans. Most of what we know about PTSD comes from studying men'.

Amara's work identifies a blind spot in trauma studies and maternity services – the overlapping of sexual assault onto birth – a silencing which she seeks to redress and resolve.

Women all over the world [...] give birth and one in three women all over the world also experience some form of sexual violence, according to the World Health Organization.

Amara concludes:

The very least we can do is make pregnancy and labour as pain free as possible for rape survivors. Considering the need, I don't understand why this hasn't been done before.

In her memoir of black British motherhood, *I Am Not Your Baby Mother,* published in 2020, best-selling author and Instagram star Candice Brathwaite gives voice to her encounter with structural racism within Britain's maternity services. The burden of trauma in birth is not borne equally. 'Feeling unwell,' Brathwaite states, of her traumatic recovery from birth, 'and not having my symptoms taken seriously was not a one-off experience'. When Brathwaite's concerns over an infected C-section were ignored by medical professionals, she entered septic shock, and was hospitalised for weeks. Why had this happened?

'In 2018,' she declares, 'some five years after Esmé was born, a report was published which helped me make sense of my experience. The MBRRACE-UK report (which is used as a tool to gather data, learn lessons and inform maternity care in the UK and Ireland) exposed the horrific statistic that, in the UK, black women are five times more likely to die in childbirth than any other race.'

Brathwaite notes, powerfully, that while the evidence contained in this report is irrefutable, 'not all are willing to believe its content':

Most healthcare professionals I have spoken to since have consistently tried to put this shocking statistic down to the fact that pregnant black women are more likely to fall prey to pregnancy-related illnesses which then lead to death. Whilst I'm not educated to speak on the science behind our bodies, I am experienced enough to attest to the fact that this is not the only reason. In my opinion, a lot of this comes down to both conscious and unconscious bias, which is in part supported by the fact that the NHS is a product of a society governed by white supremacy which is willing to uphold racist values so long as nobody blows the whistle.

Brathwaite, like Amara, is a rape survivor. Long before entering into motherhood, she spent years fighting memories of this experience. 'I told myself that I was to blame,' she writes:

> *That I shouldn't have drunk so much. That I had it coming. In doing so I underestimated the power that this experience took from me. How my sexual identity was tugged unwillingly from my own grasp and how I spent almost a decade trying to con myself into believing that I still held it in my hands. And how it was perhaps the root of my most destructive behaviour to come. I thought of all these things before the time of #MeToo.*
>
> *And by experience, I mean rape.*
>
> *There, I said it.*

Brathwaite's political writing outlines the intersectional impact of previous trauma on birth trauma – and the life-threatening friction that results when these layered traumas collide with systemic discrimination. After the difficult birth of her daughter, Brathwaite struggled with anxiety and depression. Mothering a newborn after a prolonged period of hospitalisation was 'an uphill battle'. In order to heal, Brathwaite tells us, she would have 'to get some deep therapy to unpack all the past trauma which the pressures of motherhood were now bringing to the forefront'.

Audre Lorde, in her essay 'The Transformation of Silence into Language and Action', urges us to use language to identify injustice: to designate the boundaries (the signs and signifiers) of what has universally existed but was never previously acknowledged. Brathwaite's work shares with Lorde a commitment to poetry, 'to language', as Lorde writes, 'and to the power of language, and to the reclaiming of that language which has been made to work against us'. Language, Lorde teaches us, can break silence. It can empower. It can inspire transformation. But language alone is not enough. Brathwaite moves, like Lorde, from language to action. Because what happens in birth demands more than acknowledgement: it demands change.

In September, the babies' first milk teeth came through. I showed Grace the gummy, tooth-pierced smiles, one after the other, proud of their collective effort. It has been uncomfortable for them, I said, picking one boy up to soothe him, a real battle. I remarked on the management of teething, the ever-wetting bibs, buttoned round their necks, the fretting, the fevers, the crying, the broken sleep. My pride mitigated (slightly) by the simultaneous, shocking appearance of blood, in the consulting room, on my nipples, when they bite me. The advent of teeth precipitates new ways of thinking: new ways of eating. A host of novel anxieties. Baby-led weaning? I asked Grace. Purées? Meal planning? Nutrition? Was I a bad mother if I wanted to stop breast feeding, now that they had teeth? Grace told me I should follow my heart. 'You do not need to be perfect, but good enough,' she said, referring to the paediatrician and psychoanalyst Donald Winnicott's mandate for manageable parenting goals. In 1953, Winnicott had written that the Good Enough Mother's gradual (and inevitable) failure to meet her child's needs helped her child adapt to the external reality of its environment. The child must learn that 'a mother is neither good nor bad nor the product of illusion,' Winnicott counselled, but 'a separate and independent entity'. This appealed to me. Rather than tying myself to a single mast, I pursued a medley. Carrot sticks, attacked raw, and roasted squash blended into sweet, sticky paste. The babies respond enthusiastically to the challenge. 'We have,' I laughed to Callum, when he encountered the aftermath in the kitchen, 'big eaters.'

'We do not have much time left,' Grace warned. There would only be one session with her after the birth debrief to discuss moving forward – to the next therapist, to the next chapter, to the next plan of care. Until that point, she preferred to focus on what she knew and understood: birth and babies, postnatal depression and difficulty in early motherhood. The more I spoke, the more my silence lifted. I began to notice them. The *others*. The women with the prams in the waiting room, before and after me. The names signed into the paper ledgers. *And then, and then, and then.*

With Grace's help, I put birth back together slowly. Blood was something I puzzled over often: the mystery of its origin. In my memories, the nature of the blood changed frequently. Fresh blood clotting on my children's skulls, from the forceps; the bruised lumps, angry and purple on B's skull; the scabbing wounds; the dirty dressing of my cannulas, and, of course, the lochia, the postpartum period, which streamed daily from me. The tarry blood in my bowel movements. The pink blood in my urine, and, most troubling of all, the blood that began as a greyish smear on my menstrual pad, the rancorous blood accompanied by that violent smell, flooding my body three weeks after my twins had been born.

The first night I encountered the violent smell, I told Grace, wafting up as I pulled down my underwear in the bathroom, I denied its existence. My ten-year-old sister had come to stay with us in London, and I had made her supper, listening as she described the flames on the ridgeline seen through the kitchen window, racing towards her house. There had been a bright round moon, the sky was clear and the wind fierce, the Santa Ana's running west. She declared with some vexation that she was the only one of the family to save anything useful from the fire. Before evacuating, she had gathered two blankets she had made for each of my twins in her sewing class, a teddy and a backpack full of emergency supplies for the family and pets, consisting of several tins of dog and cat food, a compass, a packet of ibuprofen and an aromatherapy diffuser to manage stress. She rescued my father's laptop and hard-drives, as he loaded dinner plates into the dishwasher, not wanting to leave a messy kitchen for the firemen who never came. My little sister told me these things as I too loaded the dishwasher and afterwards I made us each a cup of tea and we talked about the new rental, and her friends, how she was glad to be in school again: my mother had taken her to England for two months after the fire, and not provided much home education. Things were better now. 'I still struggle to read,' my sister confessed, 'and to write.' And she mentioned that her teacher had embarrassed her over this – making her read aloud in front of the class, before calling my parents and asking *why*? Now, at least, my sister had an answer. 'I can't read because I'm dyslexic,' she announced, and I was proud of her for being proud. I asked her then what the new house was like and she corrected me and said it's not my new house, it's a rental paid for by the insurance company – and then shrugged and said, 'I guess it's nice.' It was in town, and she could ride her bicycle to school and the ice-cream store and meet her friends. After we had finished eating, I took her down to the babies' nursery (my children slept in bassinets, attached to my own bed) and watched as she unpacked her bag.

Very carefully, my sister placed objects under her pillow: a crank flashlight and a compass. I asked if she always kept these nearby. 'Yeah,' she said. 'I do. Just in case, you know, there's an emergency or something.'

I spoke to Grace, then, of how my husband had brought me in the dead of night to my birth hospital, after I had collapsed naked on our bedroom floor. I told her of two women, magnificent phantoms in my memory, a midwife and a female doctor, who shimmered at my bedside, explaining that I had a uterine infection and the beginning of sepsis and that my heart had gone into a state of tachycardia – meaning that it was beating too fast, much faster than normal. These women had hooked me up to a drip and stabilised my infection. When I changed wards, the notes made in the ADU had once again been 'lost' so that when a male doctor came to visit me the next morning, he examined me for signs of uterine infection – pressing his fingers down hard, into the flesh of my groin, expecting to make me scream. He had pushed again harder, pressing his fingers into my abdomen, searching for pain, and when I did not scream, and stared blankly into space, unmoving, he turned to the audience flanking him and said with confidence: 'If she had anything in there,' he gestured to my womb, 'she would have screamed. She would have jumped a mile.' He then asked to see my engorged breasts, and opened my gown, and lifted my breasts towards the light, bare handed, and examined them with dispassion in front of his collected trainees, as one might examine a pig's cadaver in an abattoir, squeezing my nipple, bringing his face close to the areola, pinching the glands, asking if it hurt. When I said it did not hurt, he shoved his fingers once more into my abdomen and when I did not cry out in pain his frustration at my not hurting was not directed at me but at the system as a whole. He spoke to the juniors gathered around him with annoyance, saying that *she*, an unpregnant woman, did not belong here, in the birthing ward, *she* belonged in the Antenatal Day Unit, and he made this clear to the attendant midwives: this non-belonging. He wanted *this woman* out, he said, he wanted *her* gone. While he had initially suspected an infection of the mammary glands, on examining the patient's breasts, he had found no clear sign of mastitis and so would take the patient off an unnecessary course of antibiotics. Exhaustion, the burden of twins, was the cause of my delirium. The doctor treating me now addressed my husband.

'Your wife,' the doctor declared, 'is a well woman.' Callum protested at my bedside and the doctor rolled his eyes. 'You're really selling it, aren't you?' In us, he detected the clinical signs of what is termed *Twin Shock*. The parents of multiples are exhausted. They are mad, they are deluded, they are strange. 'Get some sleep,' he said to us. 'You both need it.'

Before adding, as I recall, to my husband: 'Don't be hysterical.'

Don't be hysterical. In the late 1880s, the French neurologist Jean-Martin Charcot, grandmaster of the Parisian asylum Salpêtrière, gave a public Tuesday Lecture on the subject of hysteria, or what Charcot called the 'Great Neurosis' – examining a female patient under hypnosis. He too applied pressure to a patient's womb, hoping to provoke a response.

Leaving Vienna, Freud, who had attended Charcot's lectures in Paris, took with him a small lithograph of a painting titled *A Clinical Lesson at the Salpêtrière,* which he hung above the analytical couch in his London rooms. In the lithograph, Charcot examines a hysterical, demi-conscious, bare-shouldered woman, before a sea of engrossed, dark-suited men.

I wonder what image hangs in the consulting room of the doctor who pressed his hands into my hysterogenic zones.

As soon as the doctor had uttered his own approximation of Charcot's dismissal of the hysterical condition as *a lot of noise over nothing,* he left. After him came a midwife, wheeling a trolley. She told me I would soon be allowed to go home, took out my cannula and rolled the IV apparatus away. I was relieved. I wanted to believe it was true. She measured things I did not understand. Put a clip that shone red on my finger, fit the strap on my upper arm and took my blood pressure. She was compassionate. She was kind. She placed a temperature strip gently under my arm, and noted with a smile: 'Temperature down, though you are still tachycardic.' Lying in bed, I had a resting heart rate of 134 beats per minute, generally a sign of infection. 'But you're all right,' she said warmly, 'you're doing better.' There was, of course, still the matter of the foul-smelling blood; I confessed this to her: that in the bathroom, after the doctor left, I had begun passing large, greenish clumps of mottled flesh. I had kept my dirty pad and showed this to her. She worried for a moment, looking at the blood, and then said again that discharge was normal. And anyway, the same thing, she said, happened to her, she was out walking in the playground, a few weeks after the birth of her second child, and all of a sudden, she felt terrible, she had to sit down, all this muck, she said, came right out of her, it was frightening at the time, but you know, she felt better after it cleared, much better.

Before the end of her shift that evening, the midwife

returned to say goodbye. As she spoke, she started to cry. I asked her what was wrong and she said that she'd been yelled at on the ward by another patient's husband, that a mistake had happened, not with her, with someone else, and this man had called her horrible, horrible names. She told me that she'd become a midwife because she loved the idea of ushering babies into the world, but now she questioned everything, she felt – and she used the word – *traumatised* by the system. She was not paid enough, was not thanked enough, not supported enough by this place: her shifts were endless, and there were not enough midwives to manage the patients – they were overstretched, overworked, and because of this sometimes she missed things. Awful things. She made mistakes. The mistakes made her feel terrible. And she witnessed things, things she did not know how to process: she witnessed death. She witnessed birth. She witnessed blood. And now, this evening, having witnessed all these things, she had to commute once again home on the train. She could not afford to live near the hospital, and had rented outside London, and it would take her over an hour to get home, and by the time she got back her children, whom she loved dearly, would be asleep, and she would see them only briefly in the morning, before she's back here, for another thankless shift, and she was tired, so, so, tired. No one, she felt, appreciated her. No one appreciated her existence. Not the patients, not the trust, not the government. 'I can't,' she said, hunching forward, as if struggling to bear the burden of her own weight. 'I can't do this any more. Every day I feel more and more like I'm drowning. If you could see it, what goes on in this place, if you could see what I mop off the floor, out of rooms like yours, I've seen it: other women's blood. Everywhere. Pooling in lakes. Just everywhere. Everywhere. Everywhere.'

Listed below are a number of difficult or stressful things that sometimes happen to people. For each event check one or more of the boxes to the right to indicate that (a) it happened to you personally, (b) you witnessed it happen to someone else, (c) you learned about it happening to someone close to you, (d) you were exposed to it as part of your job, (e) you're not sure if it fits or (f) it doesn't apply to you. Be sure to consider your entire life (growing up as well as adulthood) as you go through the list of events.

This Event ...

Happened to me | Witnessed it | Learned about it | Part of my job | Not sure | Doesn't apply

Number 1: Natural disaster, for example, flood, hurricane, tornado, earthquake.
Number 2: Fire and explosion.
Number 3: Transportation accident, car accident, boat accident.
Number 4: Serious accident at work, home or during recreational activity.
Number 5: Exposure to dangerous toxic substance.
Number 6: Physical assault (for example being attacked, hit, slapped, kicked, beaten up).
Number 7: Assault with a weapon.
Number 8: Sexual assault (rape, attempted rape, made

to perform any type of sexual act through force or threat of harm).

Number 9: Other unwanted or uncomfortable sexual experience.

Number 10: Combat or exposure to a war zone.

Number 11: Captivity.

Number 12: Life-threatening illness or injury.

Number 13: Severe human suffering.

Number 14: Sudden violent death (e.g. suicide, murder).

Number 15: The sudden unexpected death of someone close to you.

Number 16: Serious injury, harm or death you caused to someone else.

Number 17: Any other very stressful event or experience.

Filling in the trauma assessment forms, two years after the birth of my children, I will feel a pang of confusion: Birth Trauma and Pregnancy Loss were not individually categorised on the Life Events Checklist. This will surprise me, as miscarriage, birth and the mental illness that followed comprise one of the most traumatic sequences of events that I have lived as a woman. But it also will not surprise me. Aberrations from the accepted terrain of 'normalcy' in motherhood were not considered traumatic enough to merit categorisation. I will wonder, reading through my answers, if the absence of traumatic categories related to motherhood was accidental, an oversight, or a deliberate omission – or if the research simply hadn't caught up yet. I will write some notes in the margins to that effect and send it over to the NHS specialist managing my case.

Soon after the birth of my own children, the French writer Adélaïde Bon, herself the victim, in childhood, of a brutal rape in her leafy Parisian neighbourhood, will also confront the resurgence of traumatic memories and traumatic desires she faces on entering motherhood, in her award-winning memoir: *The Little Girl on the Ice Floe*. Bon will ask:

> *How to contain the horror in words. How to tell about the blank months. My son, my love, my darling, he might read these words one day. He will be hurt and I don't know if I will be able to fix him, to console him from that kind of hurt. But I will write these words anyway, I owe them to myself, I owe them to the little girl waiting for me on the ice floe, I owe them to all the lives of pain.*

My editor will send me a copy of Bon's book in the post, with passages dog-eared and I will read them, and feel myself seen. *This,* I will want to scribble in the margin, *this, this, this.*

Trauma elides, trauma deflects, trauma obscures. It does not want to be pinned down, and yet pin it down we must. We defeat it by rendering it milk-sodden, word-bound. We capture it with the mundane, the quotidian, the resolutely dull, the drab confessional flung into the drab, empty air. Through staccato narratives of *and then, and then, and then*, we augment, mollify, contain. We narrate it into a corner. Then and only then, can we extract the borders of what was once invisible, can we hold it and see it up close, can we own it, define it, integrate it. Once we have done this, we may find, in our possession, something else entirely: something quiet, something *still*, as Toni Morrison writes, something strong.

Understanding what had happened to me after birth, discovering the real, clinical name for my pregnancy condition, would take seven months of investigation, supported by Grace, returning to the paper records at my birth hospital with a consultant midwife, who sifted through the blow-by-blow handwritten account by the doctors who delivered me, in order to find out why I'd nearly died.

The woman who gave me the name of my birth condition dressed like a senior member of the politburo. She sat across from me in a wipe-down purple chair on the seventh or eighth floor of my birth hospital, in a small room decorated with a poster about women's reproductive health and a plastic magnolia. The consultant midwife was a highly trained expert on such things, but she seemed defeated by the time I entered her room, overwhelmed by the heaviness of what must have been a repetitive and thankless task. On the coffee table in front of her were two stacks of thick orange folders. The stack to her left had been read out before I arrived, to perhaps three or four other women, the stack to her right represented future appointments. It was clear to me, as soon as I sat down, that what we discovered, we would discover in unison. I would relive my birth via her direct mediation, observing both her boredom and her clipped surprise, putting my trust in her hands. I sat calmly in the chair in front of her, not wanting her to see my agitation, and she remarked on the weather, intractable and grey.

She then took the orange medical folder stuffed with paper notes from the top of one pile. I was surprised by the bolt of emotion that shot through me: this object had accompanied me throughout my children's gestation, it had once belonged to me, it was mine, it had lived for many months on my bedside. I had studied the scans and doctors' handwritten scrawl at different points in my journey, trying to parse meaning. I had clung to it as evidence, as proof, of the babies inside me, and I had been terrified of losing it, as it was the only thing that contained everything in one place, and was relied on heavily by specialists. In addition to my scans and growth charts, it held the handwritten notes from my delivery. The consultant midwife opened my folder and began to read with clinical detachment.

'Ah,' she said, double-checking my birthdate.

'Multiples – DCDA – Baby A cephalic (head down), Baby B transverse. Correct?'

'Yes,' I said.

Her role, I soon realised, was to assure me that what had happened could have happened no other way. She was a phantom from the Egyptian Underworld, an animal-headed figure of judgement, weighing up the scales of mothers' suffering, as I demanded ... well ... what?

A deeper understanding?

Her stance on this was clearly: no.

No silliness. No fretting.

No amount of anxiety can change the past.

I was meant to sit and listen and be illuminated by the truth as she read out the details of my delivery. Most of this information did not interest me: at this time your cervix dilated to such-and-such, at this hour you had an epidural, at this point the baby crowned. But the gist really, was: what's done is done. She was proud. She placed great confidence in the expertise of her midwifery team: its capacity to get results, to safely handle emergencies, to make split-second decisions. Forceps, ventouse, episiotomies, second-degree tears – these things she brushed aside as normal and to be expected, and I agreed. Not one of these things bothered her in the slightest. When we reached the end of my delivery she nodded to herself, and looked up at me.

'You had a good birth,' she said.

She seemed happy about this, even encouraging, and she wanted me to feel happy and encouraged too.

'Your labour,' she noted, 'lasted only eight hours, and you had a beautiful assisted delivery by the doctors, no need for an emergency caesarean. Magnificent, really. What, precisely, upset you?'

'Please,' I mumbled. 'If you don't mind, I would like to know what happened after I delivered my sons.'

I watched as the consultant midwife ran her finger down my birth notes silently, hunting for something, her glasses perched at the end of her nose.

Her brow furrowed as she searched and then she stopped.

'Ah,' she said to herself and frowned slightly before looking up: 'accreta.'

After that, the tone of our conversation changed.

'My dear,' she remarked, adjusting the glasses on her nose, 'you are exceptionally lucky.'

Placenta accreta, she explained, was an extremely rare and life-threatening maternity complication that, according to Tommy's, affects roughly 1.7 out of 10,000 pregnancies (statistics vary, and incidents of the condition have gone up in recent decades, due to higher rates of C-sections, as placenta accreta is more likely to develop on top of a pre-existing scar in the uterus). Placenta accreta spectrum impacts the cellular structure of the placenta, causing the organ to spread like a cancer, eating into the lining of the uterus, to varying degrees of severity, such that the placenta adheres to the womb and cannot dislodge after birth. The condition is a dangerous aberration of human biology, with a high morbidity rate: one in fourteen women with accreta dies. The emergency, blind removal of my own adhered placenta had caused me to haemorrhage. I had, the midwife said, lost a great deal of blood. Though she did not give me a figure, she implied I could have lost more than had been recorded in my hospital discharge notes, which at the time had been estimated at 1.6 litres. I asked the midwife, full of turmoil, after hearing all this, if I should have had a caesarean, but she brushed this aside with a terse, 'No, on the contrary, you might very well not be here.'

She asserted the following, with emphatic surety: had I had an emergency caesarean that morning – and the doctors had discovered I had placenta accreta after cutting me open – I would have had a hysterectomy on the spot, and could potentially have died, as they would not have had enough blood on hand to pump into my body to counter both my haemorrhaging and the bleeding from the caesarean.

This made me feel sick.

I'd heard the obstetrician, managing the difficult birth with intervention of my two posterior sons, saying, 'One more push and we're going in.' What if I'd had that emergency caesarean? Would I have died? The midwife did not detect my discomfort and turned her attention swiftly to the future. She warned me the accreta would likely impact my fertility, especially if the damage to my uterus had been worsened by recurrent infections – which leave scars in the uterine lining – but it was possible, she continued, to cut this scar tissue out with lasers and if the womb healed properly, I might conceive children again, though my condition left me with a high risk of infertility.

'If you find it difficult to conceive,' she added, kindly, 'we'd be happy to help you here at this hospital. We will make the best of our facilities available to you.'

I felt it then.

The anger.

The midwife, holding my birth notes, at the birth debrief, seven months after the birth of my children, pressed on at a clip. She warned me that even if I could conceive, I would never have a 'safe' or 'normal' subsequent pregnancy. That my condition carried an extremely high risk of maternal mortality – my own mortality – into the birth of any future children. According to my birth notes, when the doctor had ripped my placenta out of my body, the organ had emerged in fragments, which had been painstakingly reconstructed in a bloody puzzle. Upon finishing the reconstruction, the doctors had realised that my placenta contained ragged membranes, meaning that pieces of my placenta had stayed behind in what is known as 'retained product of conception' – leading to an increased risk of postnatal uterine infection. This too was recorded in my physical maternity file but had not been entered into my digital records. I asked the midwife how this was possible and she sighed. As information was transferred from one antiquated format to another, she presumed, a simple human error occurred: the error of accidental omission.

'All things considered,' the midwife said, 'you seem like you're doing well.'

'What do you mean, doing well?' I asked sharply.

'You're stoic. Quite stoic,' she said. 'And you're cogent. Which isn't always the case. I get the strong impression that you understand,' the consultant midwife said, with a hint of approval in her voice, 'that these things make sense to you.'

I stared at her.

Did these things make sense to me?

No.

Frankly, they did not.

Perhaps this perception of 'wellness', in my own case, could be taken as a compliment?

I told the midwife that I had worked hard over months of therapy to make peace with my suffering – but in this instance I did not feel well at all.

Sure, I felt a certain relief to be alive – yes.

I could acknowledge, too, that *yes*, the outcome might certainly have been worse.

But *doing well*?

A woman who suffers birth trauma lives with her birth every day. Relives it every day. Her 'Birth Experience' is not a pencilled note, written in haste, secreted away in an orange folder. It is not historic. It is not static. It is alive and real and present. What she *lived* is happening *now*.

Right now.

To her.

In this very room.

Throughout the first seven months of my babies' existence, I had worried, at length, about a psychological wound, hidden deep inside my uterus, a phantom of my nerves: the wreckage of a mind on fire. I blamed myself for *being* sick. For having 'poor hygiene', as one GP said. For 'not sleeping enough'. I felt guilty for inventing things, for feeling overwhelmed, for struggling to smile, for needing to lie down when I had walked too far, of hurting when I picked up my boys or played with them. Whenever I hurt, I pushed stubbornly through hurting, assuming my pain was invented. A by-product of stress and anxiety, perhaps, another secret ailment of motherhood? I held on to my belief that with the right treatment, the right therapy, the pain, which was always present – round and dull – that worsened, unpredictably – would go away. Sometimes this pain transformed into a heavy knot deep inside my pelvis, on the left side of my belly. Sometimes it shuddered up my back, yanking me down to earth. Sometimes it raged through me, in hot bursts, like an electric jolt. I was surprised when it grew narrow and deep, making it difficult to breathe. The almost constant menace of this pain contributed, deeply, to a permanent sense of frailty and unease. Would I have been less hard on myself, less angry, less ashamed by my helplessness, by my inadequacy, if I had understood the gravity of what had happened in the operating room? Would I have felt less self-loathing as a mother if I had understood the effort my body was making to recover?

Yes. Absolutely. One hundred per cent.

For months, I had battled infection after infection. Whenever a course of antibiotics ended, and my temperature spiked and I went back into hospital, I had asked myself, *why is this happening?* I had felt guilty – for inventing things, for things were out of my control – believing that I 'could not keep it together'. I had told myself that I was 'weak'. That I had 'asked for it'. Motherhood – as far as I was concerned – was about learning to live with sickness and pain. I'd discovered lots of things that nobody bothers to tell you until after you give birth, when the cultural taboo lifts and the floodgates open. Things like: breastfeeding hurts. Or: in reality, when you first meet your child, you are meeting a wild animal in a state of shock, who you have to humanise, a creature who can't tell night from day, who doesn't smile. Or that the flood of hormones in your body, after birth, as in my own case, can lead to sadness. Deep sadness. Worsened in part, by the great cultural lies I had been told throughout my pregnancy. I had no idea what an episiotomy looked like or felt like. I had no idea that because I was carrying two posterior twins a vaginal delivery would transform into a battleground – that my vagina would be cut and ripped open. I had no idea that women after a delivery like mine often aren't able to walk, if they've had what are euphemistically called 'interventions'. I had no idea that one's belly stays as swollen and full as it was before birth, for weeks, that milk doesn't come to everyone, that it's a struggle. I had no idea, until I spent weeks on postnatal wards, how much women after birth, in happiness and in despair, cry and cry. How, if we are suddenly severed from our children, our symbiotic relationship with our child, out there, alone in the world, ruptures, we fall out of control. I had discovered, in becoming a mother, a whole universe of secrets, disclosed furtively by other women, whose voices echoed in a chorus: *This happened to me, to me, to me.* While I may look, on the outside, calm and collected, internally I am a creature at war with both the past and my body. I am not, as yet, in control of my body, or what it does to me, and I feel unsettled by new information.

But this?

This winded me.

After birth, I had begged for information.

Why had I not been allowed to keep my paper maternity folder?

The one she held, primly, between officious hands?

Surely, I said to the consultant midwife, the information contained in that folder was important. The kind of information a birthing person had a right to know?

The midwife shuffled awkwardly in her seat.

The physical maternity folder, she said, did not belong to me.

It belonged to the hospital.

And then she asked if there was anything else I'd like to talk about, regarding my birth experience.

I felt my anger grow sharp.

I told the midwife that when my delivery was over, no one, not once, gave me a name for my condition or offered a reason why, no matter how many times my husband and I had pressed for answers. It took several days, I said, to receive a blood transfusion, and I was only offered one after I fainted on the ward, trying to go to the bathroom myself, when my catheter had been removed, while my husband was in the NICU with the baby I had not yet met. Nobody, I said, scanned me vaginally after my delivery. I was angry about this. I felt, intuitively, that the absence of my birth condition on my birth notes was symptomatic of a maternity system under strain. A maternity system failing mothers.

I wanted the consultant midwife to understand this anger, and so I said, when she asked if there was anything else I would like to talk about: 'Yes, actually there is.'

If losing medical notes happens once, it is a mistake. If it happens multiple times, to the same woman, in rapid succession, it is systemic.

'Perhaps,' I said to the consultant midwife, seated before her stack of orange files, 'my postnatal care at your hospital would have been managed better if two words had appeared on my hospital discharge notes: *placenta accreta*. It is not insignificant to me,' I said, 'that when a female doctor at a different hospital, twelve hours later, took the time to assess me internally she correctly diagnosed me with a uterine infection, owing to retained products of conception. Which now, looking back on it, is no surprise really.' I told the midwife that as I saw it, her hospital had made not one mistake, but several, and those mistakes had repeatedly put me at risk. To make matters worse, I said – and I named him – that male doctor's treatment of me was gendered.

The woman started in her chair: 'What do you mean gendered?'

I said: 'That doctor treated me in a gendered fashion.' *Oh, he said, speaking directly to my husband, never once addressing me. What your wife needs is a good rest.*

Look at her, he said, she looks like a well woman.

I had a life-threatening postnatal infection, after a life-threatening delivery. But that doctor had no interest in my own opinions about my own body. He had no awareness of the impact of trauma. He did not consider my capacity for dissociation. He did not examine me internally. He put his bare hands on my pubic region and pressed down. He attempted to diagnose me by hurting me: by seeing how much pain his fingers could elicit. He discounted internal evidence of infection. How many other women does this happen to? The consultant midwife at my birth debrief closed my birth file and put it to one side. She dusted off her skirt. 'It is not true,' she said, 'that this doctor who discharged you was gendered, for he loves women. Works every day to help women.' But she promised to take my points into consideration. 'I can see from your file that your case should have been handled differently. I am sorry about what happened to you. You should have been taken to our high-dependency unit after giving birth. We should have monitored you and followed up with internal scans. You should not have had to wait three days for a blood transfusion, after losing so much in the operating theatre. You should not have been discharged from our hospital again, after coming in with a uterine infection twenty-one days after birth, only to be readmitted to a different hospital, which gave you an accurate diagnosis, twelve hours later. All of this strikes me as grave cause for concern.

'We will review your case internally.'

I felt a sudden, unexpected compassion for the consultant midwife. I was wrong: she did not dress like a senior member of the politburo. She dressed like a woman under fire, protecting her own fragility with conservative tailoring. She was beleaguered by cuts to the NHS, forced to confront, day in day out, the mountain of human suffering secreted away in her dusty stack of orange maternity files. Each file belonged to a mother, or birthing partner, who would come in that day asking questions about a birth that had gone wrong. The collective trauma, manifest in that stack of paper files, must not have been easy to shoulder. How many private tragedies did those files contain? Losses that easily dwarfed my own? I looked at the midwife, and thought: *She is a good woman. She is doing her best to help.* I had asked my question and received my answer, which is as much as anyone can hope for: I would not trespass on this woman's precious time any longer. Getting up from my chair, I shook the consultant midwife's hand and thanked her for her candour and said goodbye to the little room with its stack of files and plastic magnolia and wine-coloured, wipe-clean chairs.

I walked down the corridor that led to the Antenatal Day Unit – the emergency room for expecting mothers and the birth centre on the labour ward.

I waited in the large communal entryway for the lift with a midwife and a doctor in blue scrubs, chatting about weekend plans away.

When the elevator opened a wave of women walked out, some with partners, others alone, one breathing heavily, perhaps already a few centimetres dilated, another flushed with excitement, discreetly wearing the badge of pregnancy on the lapel of her blue pea-coat. All were eager pilgrims to this place. Each on a journey of her own. The midwife had said: *I am sorry about what happened to you.*

I stepped into the elevator and was swallowed by the crowd.

'You all right?' another uniformed midwife asked, standing beside me.

'Yeah,' I said, 'I'm all right.'

Without realising it I had begun to cry. The nurse went back to her smartphone. A mother leaned into her partner, a man carrying pink balloons, their sleeping newborn snug in a car seat between them. At each floor the doors opened and at each floor, more strangers stepped in. There was a woman with an unlit cigarette dangling from her lip, wearing a pink fluffy dressing gown; an old man with round sunspots on his skin, a cannula taped to his wrist, his plastic bracelet on display, shuffling his feet in agitation on his way to pick up a paper. There was a teenage boy in a hospital wheelchair, pushed by his grandmother, or so I judged by the tenderness with which she spoke to him. We reached the ground floor. The doors pulled open and the crowd emptied into an enormous hall, more airport than hospital. I passed the cafés and bookshops and pharmacies, saw people rushing back and forth in that great testament to British socialism, the NHS. Something new settled in my body: I was grateful, in that moment, to this place, somewhere I had long vilified. Returning to it, I felt a dizzying eruption of unbounded emotion, and walked out in a blur. I trudged through blistering rain, entering a crowd, and pulled my anorak close; I thought of Eliot's *Murmur of maternal lamentation*. Reaching the Thames, I saw the boats going up and down, people walking along the riverfront, and heard in the tide a crescendo of voices, not lamenting, but resounding. Voices of women who had held me. Uniformed women, with their lanyards and gloves and gowns. Women who had saved me, pricking my skin, healing my body, women who had plunged their arms into the whirlpool, and pulled me back. I crossed a bridge before entering the Tube, as the midwife's words rang out across dark water.

You seem like you're doing well.

Perhaps this was the beginning of that statement being true?

I was grateful, then. Grateful for the communion with truth she gave me, for that sense of awakening – of giving a name to the condition that afflicted me – of coming back down into my body, of knowing *what* exactly had happened there, and why, and how, that I was not wrong to have believed that I had nearly died. Owning it brought huge reprieve. I did not know then, could not know then, that 'getting over' accreta – physically and mentally – would require years of physical healing and therapy. That when my boys turned two, my body would be assessed by doctors and I would be told not to have children again. That the risks to my life would be deemed too great. All this and more lay ahead of me. What was important, then, was simply the following: I had a *name*. And naming helped. I had not vanished as a mother. I had *survived*. I had rescued myself from silence. I would go home to my children, hold them close to my heart and express my gratitude. Gratitude for the exquisite grace they had brought to my universe, for the compassion they had shown their mother, as she battled a darkness they could not see. For the love, I choked, on that bridge, *for the love*.

'Wellness' is an idea, difficult to pin down.

I did not feel well, but I was feeling *feelings*. And feeling feelings, after living in numbness, was really something to marvel at. I felt it then: the fog lifting. The sharp pricking of cold air on my skin as the tears rolled down my cheeks, a flood unleashed after the fire. I stood on that bridge, in a throng of strangers, submitting to wave upon wave of emotion that coursed through my body like contractions.

ACKNOWLEDGEMENTS

I am deeply indebted to the National Health Service, who worked tirelessly, over two years, to ensure my family and I recovered, first from birth, and then from complications arising from Covid during the pandemic. To the others, the struggling mothers I walked beside, signing our names into worn and faded logs, as we exited and entered therapy sessions through our local Parent and Baby Units, pushing our prams: thank you. Your bravery inspired me to be brave. Rhiannon Lucy Cosslett, whip-smart, raucous, radical, bouncing my babies on your knees, you read the early drafts, and told me to keep going, damn it. Keep going. To my indomitable agent Felicity, whose encouragement carved out space for this project when I was at my most vulnerable, and to Rose, my editor at Virago, who championed the start of my career and whose vision brought life to this book: this work would not exist without you.

To the family of poets, artists, philosophers and activists that held me at university: Tina, now Tino, They/Them, Survivor, Mystic Healer, I found myself alongside you. Amin el Gamal, Alan Holt, Alex Figalho, Carlos Fonseca, Sammie Sachs, Ben Casement, Amanda Gelender, Erika Crawford, Christian Tom, Georgina Blackett, Timour Gregory, Nizar Melki,

Badawi Qawasmi. You were the light. The source. The future. To the faculty who shepherded my time as an undergraduate, and profoundly impacted my worldview: Clayborne Carson, J. Martin Evans, Roland Greene, Saikat Majumdar, Cherrie Moraga, Franco Moretti, Peggy Phelan, Tobias Wolff, Adam Zientek, thank you for teaching me the power of language. To the women who mothered me as I mothered my children: Sarah and Lucy Bellwood, Nataly Conte, Frances Costelloe, Samantha Dakin, Jessi Drewett, Gráinne Hebeler, Liane Al Ghusain, Bria Long Nabonne, Kasi Mclenaghan, Ally Stewart. You are the root, the branch, the tree. To my Ojai Crew: Carly Witt, Sarah Hartigan, Rachel Ward, Chelsea Moore, Darah and Serafina Tabrum. You taught me to be human. Dean and Cleo, Dyonne and Laurette Josiah, you shared love and flow with my family, you gifted us with hope.

Ynaiita Warjri, thank you for digging deep, and assisting research.

To the many Graces who will doubtless recognise themselves here, despite my best efforts; to Kasi, and Gráinne, who rescued me when I needed rescuing; to Líadaín Evans, who first helped me bathe my children, and later helped me write; to Callum's family, who looked after our boys, and welcomed us into their home; to my parents and siblings, who gave us strength and support: you protected us from drowning. As to you, Callum, I am alive, today, in no small part, due to your daily acts of love. I am grateful, also, to a generation of survivors who have broken silence, and led by example, giving me, and countless others, the courage to speak out. Today, finishing this, I am feeling better, but perhaps, tomorrow, I will not. That is okay. It is okay *not* to feel better. It is okay *not* to produce art. There is so much pressure, in narrative, for us to 'recover', to reach 'catharsis', to find 'resolution', to 'speak out'. I offer resolution here because I have found it, but that resolution is as much truth as sleight of hand, a conjuring trick. I may never manage to 'resolve' what has happened to me. In naming it, I have learned to live with it, and this in turn breaks a pattern of suffering. Naming is, for me, a magical act: it is a way of saying daily, *I am alive*. I have harnessed naming to bring order to chaos. Naming maps experience into history. Contains, within it, a legacy and a lineage: it offers up a spectrum of thought. But naming cannot undo what was done.

Hope, for me, is found in the telling.

NOTES

DEDICATION

The nurses give back my clothes Plath, S., 'Three Women', *Collected Poems* (London: Faber, 1981), p. 183

AFTERBIRTH

Time is short and full Dickinson, E., 'Letter to Mrs. J. G. Holland, about September 1880', reproduced in T. Olsen, *Mother to Daughter, Daughter to Mother: Mothers on Mothering, a reader and diary* (London: Virago, 1985), p. 201

Privilege saturates Nelson, M., *The Argonauts* (London: Melville House, 2016), p. 121

A woman is a ritual Lim, G., 'Wonder Woman', *This Bridge Called My Back: Writings of Radical Women of Color*, 2nd edition (New York: Kitchen Table, Women of Color Press, 1983), p. 26

In Lucania, there is de Martino, E., 'Binding and mother's milk', *Magic: A theory from the South*, translated by Zinn, D.L., (Chicago: Hau Books, University of Chicago Press, 2001), p. 43–44 *a stowaway* Ingram, P., *A Year in the Castle* (Laurel Books, 2020)

'Celeb moms who ate their placentas', *Parents.com* (4 March 2015), https://www.parents.com/parenting/celebrity-parents/moms-dads/placentas/

Placenta, placenta, placenta Nelson, F., 'Gaby Hoffmann: Why I Ate My Placenta', *People* (6 Jan 2015), https://people.com/parents/gaby-hoffmann-girls-premiere-placenta-encapsulation/

I'm having it freeze-dried Fisher, K., 'Kim Kardashian Reveals Plans to Eat Her Placenta', *Eonline* (14 December 2015), https://www.eonline.com/news/723850/kim-kardashian-reveals-plans-to-eat-her-placenta

Every time I take a pill Kimble, L., 'Kim Kardashian West Is Taking Placenta Pills Again: I Had No "Signs of Depression" After North's Birth', People.com (3 December 2020), https://people.com/parents/kim-kardashian-west-eating-placenta-pills-avoid-postpartum-depression/

My doctor had to stick Beck, L., '9 Things Kim Kardashian Said About How Hard Pregnancy Really Is', *Cosmopolitan* (5 December 2015), https://www.cosmopolitan.com/entertainment/celebs/news/a50353/things-kim-kardashian-said-during-pregnancy/

Without any scientific evidence Farr, A., et al., 'Human placentophagy: a review', *American Journal of Obstetrics and Gynecology*, 218/4 (2018), 401, https://www.ajog.org/article/S0002-9378(17)30963-8/fulltext

pregnancy is above all de Beauvoir, S., *The Second Sex*, translated by C. Borde and S. Malovany-Chevallier (London: Vintage, 2011), pp. 551–2

Psychological trauma Herman, J., *Trauma and Recovery*, 3rd edition (New York: Basic Books, 1992), p. 33

I am sick today Akiko, Y., 'Labour Pains', *Ain't I A Woman! Poems by Black and White Women* (London: Virago Press, 1987), pp. 76–7

inextricably involved Foucault, M., *Madness and Civilization: A History of Insanity in the Age of Reason* (London: Tavistock Publications Limited, 1967)

the brain suffers together Green, M. H., *The Trotula: An English Translation of the Medieval Compendium of Women's Medicine* (Philadelphia: University of Pennsylvania Press, 2002), p. 86

nuns, and more ancient maids Burton, R., 'Symptoms of Maids', Nuns' and Widows' Melancholy' in *The Anatomy of Melancholy* (New York: New York Review of Books, 2001), p. 415

Complain many times Burton, p. 415

angorem animi Burton, p. 416

Many of them cannot tell Burton, p. 416

I feel as though Gilman, C. P., 'Correspondence from Charlotte Perkins Gilman to Martha Allen Luther Lane, July 8, 15, 1885', *Charlotte Perkins Gilman Papers*, D.513, Rare Books, Special Collections, and Preservation, River Campus Libraries, University of Rochester. Accessed via the University's digital collections: https://digitalcollections.lib.rochester.edu/ur/correspondence-charlotte-perkins-gilman-martha-allen-luther-lane-july-8-15-1885-3

Do publish those letters Woolf quoted by Gloden Dallas in her introduction to *Maternity: Letters from Working Women* (London: Virago, 1978)

The notion that pain Davies, M. L. , *Maternity: Letters from Working Women* (London: Virago, 1978), pp. 3–4

It is lack of knowledge Davies, p. 33

the baby was a fine Davies, p. 40

A miscarriage followed Davies, pp. 44–5

I do hope you do not feel Davies, p. 167

Perhaps what goes by the name Rose, J., *Mothers: An Essay on Love and Cruelty* (London: Faber & Faber, 2018), p. 185

TALKING CURE

In motherhood a woman Cusk, R., *A Life's Work: On Becoming a Mother*, 2nd ed (London: Faber & Faber, 2001), p. 9

I go to slay my children Euripides, *The Medea*, translated by Murray G., M.A., L.L.D. (New York: Oxford University Press, 1906), p. 68

When the creature was twenty Kempe, M., *The Book of Margery Kempe*, translated and edited by B. A. Windeatt, 2nd edition (London: Penguin, 2019), p. 11

What eylith þe woman Middle English original given as context in the British Library's online introduction to the medieval paper codex of *The Book of Margery Kempe*, (Shelfmark: Add MS 61823), https://www.bl.uk/collection-items/the-book-of-margery-kempe

devils opening their mouths Kempe, p. 12

of good esteem for godliness Winthrop, J., *The History of New England, 1630-1649.* (Boston: Phelps and Farnham, 1825), p. 279

the maternal heart of darkness Rich, A., *Of Woman Born:*

Motherhood as Experience and Institution, 2nd edition (New York: W.W. Norton & Company, 1986), p. 256

neurotypical bias Wang, E. W., 'Diagnosis', *The Collected Schizophrenias* (London: Penguin Books, 2019), p. 4

I come back, as we must Rich, pp. 277–8

into a demon's face Cho, C., *Inferno: A Memoir of Motherhood and Madness*, 2nd edition (London: Bloomsbury, 2020), p. 183

felt like I'd Cho, p. 186

There, I thought Cho, p. 62

Someone who has seen a house collapse Ginzburg, N., 'The Son of Man' in *The Little Virtues* (London: Daunt Books, 2018), p. 80

is a vital necessity Lorde, A., 'Poetry is Not a Luxury', *Sister Outsider* (London: Penguin Classics, 2019), p. 26

poetry is the way we help Lorde, p. 26

THEORETICAL ISSUES

The task of calling things Solnit, R., 'A Short History of Silence', *The Mother of All Questions* (London: Granta, 2017), p. 66

Death, danger, sickness, losses Hutchinson, L., *Order and Disorder*, edited by D. Norbrook (New Jersey: John Wiley and Sons, 2001)

often quoted to describe hooks, b., *Feminist Theory: from margin to centre* (Boston: South End Press, 1984), p. 1–2

The inexperience of her youth Pliny the Younger, 'Epistle X: Pliny to Fabatus' *The Epistles of Pliny the Younger: Translated from the Original Latin with Explanatory Notes*, Vol II (Edinburgh: A. Donaldson & J. Reid, 1762), p. 74

The time had now come Sander, N., *Rise and Growth of the Anglican Schism* (London: Burns and Oates, 1887), p. 132

It is a subject for pity Pliny the Elder, 'Book VII, Chapter 5 (6) Indications of the Sex of the Child during the pregnancy of the mother', *The Natural History*, translated by John Bostock, M.D., F.R.S., and H.T. Riley, Esq., B.A., (London: Taylor and Francis, 1855), accessed through the *Perseus Digital Library Project* at Tufts University, http://www.perseus.tufts.edu

Dream that my little baby Shelley, M. W. G., 'Entry of 19 March 1815', *The Journals of Mary Shelley 1814-1844: Volume 1: 1814-1822*, edited by Paula R. Feldman and Diana Scott Kilvert (Oxford: Oxford University Press, 1987), p. 70

a new study For a more detailed examination, see Farren, J., et al. 'Posttraumatic stress, anxiety and depression following miscarriage and ectopic pregnancy: a multicenter, prospective, cohort study' *American Journal of Obstetrics and Gynecology*, 222/4 (2020), p. 367.E1-367.E22, https://pubmed.ncbi.nlm.nih.gov/31953115/

those with significant Professor Bourne interviewed by Kate Wighton in 'Miscarriage and ectopic pregnancy may trigger symptoms of post traumatic stress disorder', *Imperial College London* (15 Jan. 2020), https://www.imperial.ac.uk/news/194715/miscarriage-ectopic-pregnancy-trigger-long-term-post-traumatic/

a smaller pilot study Farren, J., et al., 'Post-traumatic stress, anxiety and depression following miscarriage or ectopic pregnancy: a prospective cohort study', *BMJ Open*, 6/11 (2 November 2016), bmjopen.bmj.com/content/6/11/e011864

At the moment Farren makes these comments in an article titled 'Early miscarriage and ectopic pregnancy may trigger post-traumatic stress disorder', *Tommy's* (2 November 2016), https://www.tommys.org/about-us/charity-news/early-miscarriage-and-ectopic-pregnancy

CASE HISTORY

A diagnosis is comforting Wang, E. W., 'Diagnosis', *The Collected Schizophrenias* (London: Penguin Books, 2019), p. 5

The conflict between Herman, J., *Trauma and Recovery*, 3rd edition (New York: Basic Books, 1992), p. 1

INNATE DISPOSITION

I am angry Alcott, L. M., *Little Women* (Boston: Little, Brown and Company, 1915), p. 99

da Vinci, L., 'The foetus in the womb; sketches and notes on reproduction c.1511', from the *Corpus of Anatomical Drawings* held in the Royal Collection of HM Queen Elizabeth II. Facsimile via the Royal Collection Trust's digital archive: https://www.rct.uk/collection/919102/the-fetus-in-the-womb-sketches-and-notes-on-reproduction

In this child Clayton, M., and Philo, R., *Leonardo da Vinci: Anatomist* (London: Royal Collection Enterprises, 2012)

Hysterics suffer Breuer, J., and Freud, S., *Studies in Hysteria*, translated by N. Lockhurst (London: Penguin Classics, 2004), p. 11

Future, past, future Moretti, F., *Modern Epic: The World System from Goethe to García Márquez*, translated by Q. Hoare (New York: Verso, 1995), p. 242

narratively interesting Moretti, p. 243

The body in pain Eckstein, B., 'The Body, the Word, and the State: J. M. Coetzee's '"Waiting for the Barbarians"', *NOVEL: A Forum on Fiction*, Duke University Press, 22/2 (1989), pp. 175–98, https://doi.org/10.2307/1345802

I see her Coetzee, J. M., *Waiting for the Barbarians* (London: Vintage, 2004), p. 163

But with this woman Coetzee, p. 46

It appears to me impossible Wollstonecraft, M., and Godwin, W., *A short residence in Sweden, Norway and Denmark, and Memoirs of the Author of the 'The Rights of Woman'*, edited by R. Holmes, (Middlesex: Penguin Classics, 1987), p. 112

TIME-LINING

I have been told Morrison, T., *Mouth Full of Blood: Essays, Speeches, Meditations* (London: Chatto & Windus, 2019)

Stillness Morrison, 2019

People never speak Barthes, R., 'Some notes on Maman', *Mourning Diary*, translated by Howard, R. (New York: Hill and Wang, 2012), p. 251

Psychoanalysis in the hands Berman, J., *The Talking Cure: Literary Representations of Psychoanalysis* (New York: New York University Press, 1985), p. 4

In this part of the world Krishnamurti, J., 'Ojai, 41st Entry, 8th

April 1975', *Krishnamurti's Journal* (San Francisco: Harper and Row, 1982), p. 89

have an undying faith van der Kolk, B., *The Body Keeps the Score* (London: Penguin Books, 2015), p. 231

immediately and permanently Breuer, J., and Freud, S., 'The Physical Mechanisms of Hysterical Phenomena', in J. Strachey's *The Standard Edition of the Complete Psychological Works of Sigmund Freud* (London: Hogarth Press, 1893), reproduced in van der Kolk, *The Body Keeps the Score*, p. 231

that at the bottom Freud, S., 'The Aetiology of Hysteria' in J. Strachey's *The Standard Edition of the Complete Psychological Works of Sigmund Freud* (London: Hogarth Press, 1962) p. 203. Quoted by Elaine Westerlund in her article 'Freud on Sexual Trauma: An Historical Review of Seduction and Betrayal', *Psychology of Women Quarterly*, 10/ 4 (December 1986), pp. 297–310. See also: Herman, *Trauma and Recovery*, p. 13

I am as isolated Masson, J. M., 'Freud and the Seduction Theory: A challenge to the foundations of psychoanalysis' *The Atlantic*, (February 1984), https://www.theatlantic.com/magazine/archive/1984/02/freudand-the-seduction-theory/376313/?utm_source=email&utm_medium=social&utm_campaign=share
See also: Herman's succinct analysis of Freud's abandonment of Seduction Theory in 'A Forgotten History', *Trauma and Recovery*.

the unspeakable tragedy Sassoon, S., *The Complete Memoirs of George Sherston* (London: Faber & Faber, 1971), p. 557. See also: Morris, D. J., *The Evil Hours: A Biography of Post-Traumatic Stress Disorder*, frontispiece. Reproduced in Herman, *Trauma and Recovery*, p. 23

Strecker, E.A., M.D., and Ebaugh, F.G., M.D., 'Psychoses occurring during the puerperium', *American Medical Association*, 15/2

(1926), pp. 239-252, accessed online via the JAMA Network's Archives of Neurology and Psychiatry. https://jamanetwork.com/journals/archneurpsyc/article-abstract/643490

Zilboorg, G., 'The dynamics of schizophrenic reactions related to pregnancy and childbirth', *American Journal of Psychiatry* (January 1929) Vol 85, Issue 4 pp. 733-67

analogy between parturition Rose, J., *Mothers: An Essay on Love and Cruelty* (London: Faber & Faber, 2018), p. 49

They, men, allege Euripides, *Medea*, translated by Oliver Taplin, *Euripides I*, ed. D. Greene and R. Lattimore (Chicago: University Press, 2013), 250-53, II. 1091-1116, reproduced in Rose, *Mothers*, p. 49

had shorter gestation periods Paffenbarger, R. S., 'Epidemiological Aspects of Parapartum Mental Illness', *British Journal of Preventive & Social Medicine*, 18/4 (1964), pp. 189-95

speaking to my ob/gyn Sanford, W., 'Formative Years: The Birth of *Our Bodies Ourselves*', Sanford recalled how postpartum depression led her to the Women's Health Movement in 1969, speaking alongside Joan Ditzion, Nancy Miriam Hawley, and Paula Doress-Worters, all co-founders of the Boston Women's Health Collective, during a panel at a conference organised by the Women's, Gender, & Sexuality Studies Program at Boston University, titled *A Revolutionary Moment: Women's Liberation in the late 1960s and early 1970s* (March 27 to 29 2014). Transcript available via *Our Bodies, Ourselves*, https://www.ourbodiesourselves.org/wp-content/uploads/2020/06/Ditzion-Formative-Years-The-Birth-of-Our-Bodies-Ourselves.pdf

Terra incognita Brockington interviewed by Glangeaud, N., in the 'History of the Marcé Society (1980-2016)', *Marcé Society* (1 September 2016), https://marcesociety.com/wp-content/uploads/

2013/11/Marce-Society-History-1980-2016_nine_1September2016.pdf

Someone compared Glangeaud, 2016

I [had come] across a small Beck, C. T., Driscoll, J. W., and Watson, S., *Traumatic Childbirth* (Abingdon: Routledge, 2013), p. 2

An event occurring Beck, C. T., 'Birth Trauma: in the eye of the beholder', *Nursing Research*, 53, 28–35, reproduced in Beck, *Traumatic Childbirth*, p. 8

I felt like Beck, et al., *Traumatic Childbirth*, p. 9

The experiences of women Kitzinger, S., *Birth Crisis* (New York: Routledge, 2006), p. 69

trust your body Simpkin, P., and Klaus, P., *When Survivors Give Birth: understanding and healing the effects of early sexual abuse on childbearing women* (Seattle, WA: Classic Day Publishing, 2004), p. 74, reproduced in Beck, *Traumatic Childbirth*, p. 39

re-traumatization taking place Beck, et al., *Traumatic Childbirth*, p. 40

postpartum PTSD deserves special mention Simpkin and Klaus, *When Survivors Give Birth*, p. 394

Last year I met Amara, P., 'Pregnancy and Birth can be dangerously traumatic for Rape Victims. Now I've found a way to help', *Independent* (10 June 2016), https://www.independent.co.uk/voices/pregnancy-and-birth-can-be-dangerously-traumatic-rape-victims-i-ve-found-way-help-them-a7073976.html

Despite the fact that rape Morris, D. J., *The Evil Hours: A Biography of Post-Traumatic Stress Disorder* (New York: First Mariner Books, 2016), p. 64

Women all over the world Amara, 2016

Feeling unwell Brathwaite, C., *I Am Not Your Baby Mother* (London: Quercus, 2020), p. 123

not all are willing to believe its content Brathwaite, p. 124

I told myself Brathwaite, p. 46

to language, and to the power Lorde, A., 'The Transformation of Silence into Language and Action', *Sister Outsider* (London: Penguin Classics, 2019), p. 32

a mother is neither good Winnicott, D.W., 'Mirror-role of the mother and family in child development', in P. Lomas' edition of *The predicament of the family: a psycho-analytical symposium* (London: Hogarth Press, 1967), pp. 26–33

a lot of noise Goetz, C., *Charcot the Clinician: The Tuesday Lessons. Excerpts from Nine Case Presentations on General Neurology Delivered at the Salpêtrière Hospital in 1887-88* (New York: Raven Press, 1987), pp. 104-5, reproduced in Herman, *Trauma and Recovery*, p. 11

Listed below Weathers, F.W., et al., *The PTSD Checklist for DSM-5 (PCL-5)*, 2013. The scale, developed by the US Government's National Center for PTSD, is used for diagnostic trauma assessment within the NHS. See: https://www.ptsd.va.gov/professional/assessment/documents/PCL5_LEC_criterionA.PDF

How to contain Bon, A., *The Little Girl on the Ice Floe*, translated by R. Diver, 2nd edition (London: MacLehose Press, 2020), p. 134

affects roughly 1.7 out of 10,000 'Placenta accreta explained', *Tommy's*, Pregnancy Hub, Blogs and Stories (23 June 2017), https://www.tommys.org/pregnancy-information/blogs-and-stories/im-pregnant/pregnancy-news-and-blogs/placenta-accreta-explained

Murmur of maternal lamentation Eliot, T. S., 'The Wasteland', *Poetry Foundation*, https://www.poetryfoundation.org/poems/47311/the-waste-land